SUPERHEALTH

Dr Payne is a General Practitioner working in Solihull, who has been practising Environmental Medicine since 1979. He has a second career as a writer and broadcaster making frequent radio and TV appearances and regularly producing articles for a wide variety of magazines and newspapers. He is also interested in the use of computers in medicine and has designed the CADTEMP program (Computer Aided Diagnosis and Treatment of Environmental Medical Problems) and 'The Toxic Doomsday Book and Calendar'.

SUPERHEALTH

An Introduction to Environmental Medicine

Dr Mark Payne

MA (Oxon) MB BS (London) MRCS LRCP (London)

Thorsons
An Imprint of HarperCollins*Publishers*

Thorsons
An Imprint of HarperCollins*Publishers*
77–85 Fulham Palace Road,
Hammersmith, London W6 8JB

Published by Thorsons 1992
10 9 8 7 6 5 4 3 2 1

© Mark Payne 1992

Mark Payne asserts the moral right to
be identified as the author of this work

A catalogue record for this book
is available from the British Library

ISBN 0 7225 2589 3

Printed in Great Britain by
The Bath Press, Bath, Avon

CONTENTS

To Kelly, David and John

ACKNOWLEDGEMENTS

In Environmental Medicine and its predecessor, Clinical Ecology, it is important to acknowledge that progress has occurred only because almost all the pioneers have suffered from 'allergic' illness themselves, and have been forced to find cures due to personal suffering. Just as, in the case of architecture, if architects lived in the buildings they designed they would almost certainly design some of them very differently, so in medicine, patients are completely justified in having more confidence in doctors who have shared their experiences.

There is a further important message to be acknowledged and acted upon by the contemporary medical system. The message is that if doctors are unable to look after themselves (the profession has high rates of suicide and alcholism), their families (high rates of suicide, alcoholism and divorce), and their colleagues (junior hospital doctors are still forced to work 70–120 hours a week), then they are not in a suitable position successfully to advise patients about health and treatment of disease.

I would like to thank Dr Norman Bertenshaw for advice on engineering concepts, Dr Jean Monro for her vision of Environmental Medicine, my good friends Rolf Norfolk, Eddie Holland, Roy and Virginia Ronnie, and Desmond and Sheila Martin for their support. Also my researcher Donna Jackson, my partner Dr Keith Gent, and my wife Lynn for her endless enthusiasm, support and valuable suggestions. Finally, a special mention must go to Margaret Shepheard who has, once again, put in many hours and managed to turn hieroglyphics into a high quality manuscript.

FOREWORD: ENVIRONMENTAL MEDICINE — THE KEY TO OUR FUTURE HEALTH

We are fortunate that there are now many distinguished groups and individuals committed to repairing the ecological damage to the planet caused by our 20th century production of contaminants. International initiatives are being arranged to reverse the 'greenhouse effect', loss of the tropical rain-forests, and destruction of the ozone layer. Without being complacent, best guesstimates suggest that with a little luck these initiatives may achieve the desired effect.

Unfortunately, a far more profound and largely under-recognized danger to all our futures is already looming very large on the horizon. This danger is the emergence of environmentally-induced diseases, which are now becoming so widespread that they affect the quality of life of almost every person in the western world. These diseases range from vague symptoms like 'feeling tired all the time', often mistakenly attributed to virus infections, through eczema, asthma, migraine, colitis and even some forms of cancer.

The main treatable cause of these diseases is the widespread pollution of air, food, and water. City air is now routinely contaminated by traffic exhausts, petrochemicals, form-aldehyde and other combustion fumes. Most food and tap water has unacceptably high levels of additives, pesticides and other toxic chemicals.

There is a high health cost to be paid for overloading our bodies with these toxic substances, namely an explosion in environmentally-induced diseases, whose incidence is now between two and ten times higher than it was at the time of World War II.

Having stated the problem, it is reassuring that we already have the solution in Environmental Medicine, which inescapably will become the healthcare philosophy of the 21st century. The theories of Environmental Medicine have already been worked out, but our main task now is that of communicating this information to the population. Our urgent mission is to spread the message to enough doctors and patients within the next five years in order to stem the epidemic of environment-ally-induced diseases. The fact that you are reading this is the first step on the road to knowledge, and I hope that you are soon embracing the principles of Environmental Medicine as a routine part of your life.

Professor William Rea
World's first Professor in Environmental Medicine, Director of the Environmental Health Centre, Dallas, Texas, March 1992

INTRODUCTION

If someone told you that there was now a new form of medical care that could probably offer you:

- A feeling of positive well being
- An increase in your energy levels
- An improvement in concentration and memory
- A relatively easy way to get down to your ideal weight
- A way to sleep well at night and wake up refreshed
- A way to control and sometimes cure common allergic illness like eczema, asthma, migraine and colitis

then you'd certainly be interested.

Well, in many cases these things are now possible – by using the emerging science of Environmental Medicine.

The natural state of your body is health, and if you're ill then it usually means that you're making a mistake in some aspect of your life, for example your diet, your job, your housing, your hobbies or your social situation. Environmental Medicine looks at all these areas in order to identify the factors that may be giving you the problem. When adverse factors are removed, and adequate vitamins and mineral supplements given, the disease process can often be reversed, with a return to positive health.

Environmental Medicine has five basic tenets. Although conventional medicine claims to follow some of these principles, they are applied by most practitioners of Environmental Medicine in a completely committed way.

THE HOLISTIC PRINCIPLE

In common with other forms of alternative medicine, Environmental Medicine comes to a diagnosis on the basis of the *total symptom picture*, rather than looking merely at one organ. It then produces a treatment plan based on your lifestyle (diet, occupation, housing, hobbies and social situation). In contrast, conventional medicine has a much narrower approach and tends to concentrate on one symptom. Most of the effort is spent investigating a *single* organ to come to a diagnosis. Once a diagnosis has been made, the treatment is usually to take drugs for that single organ, and there is little attention to the rest of the body and lifestyle.

THE PREVENTIVE PRINCIPLE

Environmental Medicine hopes to *prevent* illnesses from occurring, or else treat them at a very early stage by removing the environmental causes of those illnesses. The majority of chronic diseases are at least partially predictable. They occur because of a problem of lifestyle, for example a junk-food diet, exposure to chemicals at work, smoking, excess drinking, housing or hobbies filled with environmental hazards, or a stressful home life. However, the progress of most diseases is reversible if caught early. The body has an amazing ability to heal itself providing that the lifestyle problems causing the illness are removed. In order to get better, positive lifestyle change is essential.

THE PATIENT-POWER PRINCIPLE

Information is power, and the quality of your decisions is dependent on the quality of your information. A fundamental tenet of Environmental Medicine is to give you far more information and, therefore, control over your own health. The vast majority of Environmental Medicine does not require the use of any drugs or medication, rather the removal of all environmental factors causing illness. In most cases, a dramatic improvement in your health can be achieved by making these changes. Environmental Medicine does, however, require active patient participation, so that you take responsibility for your own health. This means altering your lifestyle to get rid of disease-promoting factors rather than just expecting to pop a pill.

THE RESOURCE MANAGEMENT PRINCIPLE

The basis of the green movement is sensible management of the world's limited resources to ensure continued survival and health of all plant and animal species. The basis of Environmental Medicine is the sensible management of the *individual's* limited resources to try to gain the best possible health. Environmental Medicine is seeking to reverse the alarming finding that people with fewer resources (time, money, education, family support) die younger and suffer from more illnesses. If the *existing* knowledge about disease-causing factors and their treatment is properly used, then better health and life expectancy are likely to follow.

THE SOCIAL CHANGES PRINCIPLE

It is sometimes said 'An electorate gets the Government that it deserves' and 'Governments are as bad as they dare'. Most health-related problems in the world are *political* rather than technological. The technologies to give the population clean food and water supply, sanitation, education, reasonable housing, transport and work conditions have been available since Roman times. Radical improvements in health care will not occur until there are improvements in the political and social system.

PART I

AN INTRODUCTION TO ENVIRONMENTAL MEDICINE

CHAPTER ONE

BASIC PRINCIPLES OF ENVIRONMENTAL MEDICINE

Here is some bad news, and some good news. The bad news:

the twentieth Century is making you ill! Six out of every ten people attending their GP are suffering from symptoms and diseases (often loosely called 'allergies') *directly* caused by the twentieth Century way of living.

The good news:

Environmental Medicine has a very good chance of getting you back to health by removing the cause of these problems.

Now read on . . .

A study of patients attending their family doctor revealed that.

- 3 out of 10 have symptoms exclusively due to 'allergy';
- 3 out of 10 have symptoms partially due to 'allergy';
- The remaining 4 out of 10 have symptoms unrelated to 'allergy'.

WHAT IS 'ALLERGY'?

An allergy is a reaction to a 'foreign' substance (a neo-toxin or a poison of the twentieth century). This is using the original definition coined by Von Pirquet in 1906, which means an altered reaction (*alter* meaning other, *ergon* meaning reaction). This reaction may occur at

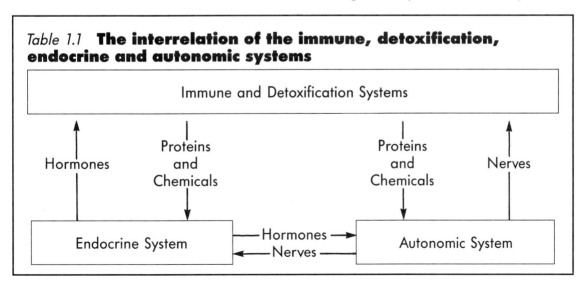

Table 1.1 **The interrelation of the immune, detoxification, endocrine and autonomic systems**

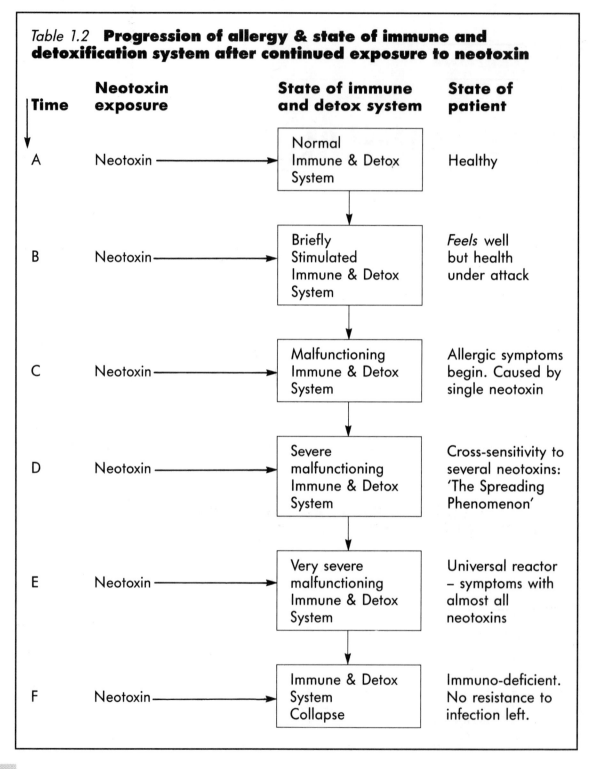

Table 1.2 **Progression of allergy & state of immune and detoxification system after continued exposure to neotoxin**

↓Time	Neotoxin exposure	State of immune and detox system	State of patient
A	Neotoxin ⟶	Normal Immune & Detox System	Healthy
B	Neotoxin ⟶	Briefly Stimulated Immune & Detox System	*Feels* well but health under attack
C	Neotoxin ⟶	Malfunctioning Immune & Detox System	Allergic symptoms begin. Caused by single neotoxin
D	Neotoxin ⟶	Severe malfunctioning Immune & Detox System	Cross-sensitivity to several neotoxins: 'The Spreading Phenomenon'
E	Neotoxin ⟶	Very severe malfunctioning Immune & Detox System	Universal reactor – symptoms with almost all neotoxins
F	Neotoxin ⟶	Immune & Detox System Collapse	Immuno-deficient. No resistance to infection left.

any time after the first exposure, when the 'foreign' substance may enter the body through the mouth (eating or drinking), lungs (inhaled), or skin (contact with skin). The unpleasant reaction is produced by the immune system and a failure of the detoxification system. The immune system is composed of white cells and antibodies which both circulate in the blood. The detoxification system is composed of enzymes occurring in every cell of the body, but especially in the liver. The immune system is controlled by hormones (like adrenalin and hydrocortisone), and these have a large effect on the autonomic system, which works automatically and controls essential functions like breathing, heart rate, function of bowels and bladder. The enzymes of the detoxification system break down foreign substances that enter the body, and excrete them either through the liver (faeces), kidneys (urine), skin (sweat) or sexual secretions (see Table 1.1).

The normal function of the immune system is to inspect all substances entering the body and decide whether they are harmless (for example organic foods), or harmful (for example bacteria, viruses, fungi and parasites). People with allergies have a defective immune system, which wrongly identifies harmless molecules as harmful intruders, and/or a defective immune system which is unable to get rid of the offending substances. The immune system also overreacts to chemicals and pollutants (neotoxins) giving rise to a wide variety of poorly defined symptoms which may affect any of the body systems and often several systems simultaneously (e.g. headache, arthritis, colitis).

The presence of a foreign substance or neotoxin briefly causes a heightened sensitivity, which stimulates the immune system and detoxification system to work harder. The immune system works harder by producing antibodies, many sorts of proteins, and extra white cells. The detoxification system works harder by producing more enzymes, a process termed *adaption* (B). (B) is then replaced by (C), in which malfunctioning immune and detoxification systems give allergic symptoms to a single neotoxin (e.g. formaldehyde). If neotoxin exposure continues (D), the immune and detoxification systems become much less discriminating, and a 'spreading phenomenon', occurs in which there is a cross-sensitivity to many chemicals and substances. The immune and detoxification systems react to any neotoxin that has a chemical similarity to the initial one. If exposure continues (E) the immune and detoxification systems begin to respond adversely to almost everything (e.g. most foods, and chemicals), and the person becomes a 'universal reactor'. If exposure to the neotoxin continues, the immune and detoxification systems go into a state of collapse (F) and the patient has little or no resistance left to any infection (see Table 1.2).

WHAT CAUSES ALLERGIES?

Allergies are caused by *neotoxins*, which are poisons of the 20th century. A neotoxin is a very broad term used to describe any sort of harmful agent which may cause an environmentally induced illness, often called an 'allergy', in a susceptible individual. The sources of allergies are:

- **Biological:** Food and drink, bacterial, viral and fungal infections, and parasites, animal and plant proteins;
- **Chemical:** A vast range including petrochemicals, pesticides, toxic metals;
- **Physical:** Electromagnetic radiation (e.g. radio, microwaves and X-rays), sound and vibrations, geopathic stress;

Allergies Are cont'd (handwritten)

free radicals (handwritten margin note)

● **Mental:** Stress.

The term allergy is a very loose one, but the mechanism occurring in most allergies is that neotoxins cause production of excess 'free radicals' within cells. Free radicals are atoms or molecules with a positive or negative charge due to one or more unpaired outer electrons, for example a hydrogen atom, molecular oxygen, or metals such as iron or copper. Free radicals are essential for cells to release energy and are only destructive when they become present in excess numbers. They are removed by the detoxification system, that is anti-oxidant enzymes (superoxide dismutase), and antioxidant vitamins (A, C and E).

Biological, chemical, physical and mental neotoxins are all able to produce excess free radicals which then overwhelm the cell's antioxidant capacity. If free radicals are not removed then they may start a chain reaction causing a cascade of further toxic products. The free radicals can cause major damage to cells by:

● Attacking the fats in cell membranes causing them to become more permeable and let in substances that are usually kept out;
● Attacking proteins including enzymes and DNA, stopping them from working properly;
● Altering glucose metabolism so that toxic substances are produced.

Allergies develop when free radicals are produced faster than the detoxification system's ability to remove them. The accumulated free radicals (the *Total Load of Neotoxins*) cause the tissue damage and breakdown in function called allergy.

WHY ARE ALLERGIES MUCH MORE COMMON NOW THAN FORTY YEARS AGO?

Most allergies are between two and ten times more common than they were forty years ago. There are three basic reasons for this massive change:

● The vastly increased load of chemical neotoxins in air, food and water. Pollution of air, food and water causes neotoxins to build up (bioaccumulate) in the body and when the *Total Load* gets above the threshold for illness an allergy occurs;
● Vastly increased indoor air pollution as a result of modern building methods. Modern buildings are made using materials that give off lots of toxic chemicals, especially formaldehyde. The buildings are made airtight, and the greatly reduced ventilation does not allow chemicals to escape.
● Modern production methods yield food that is deficient in essential nutrients such as vitamins, minerals, and essential fatty acids (EFAs).

HOW CAN I TELL IF I'M SUFFERING FROM AN ALLERGY?

Chronic allergic illnesses are very common, and sufferers will almost always have at least one of the six symptoms in the list below; tick the relevant box if you suffer from any of the symptoms. If you have one of the symptoms in the list, although you are likely to be allergic, it is important for your doctor to rule out other causes such as anaemia or thyroid disease. If you have three or more symptoms, you are almost certainly allergic. You may notice that your symptoms come on after exposure to a particular neotoxin, and that is the substance that is very likely to be the one causing your problem.

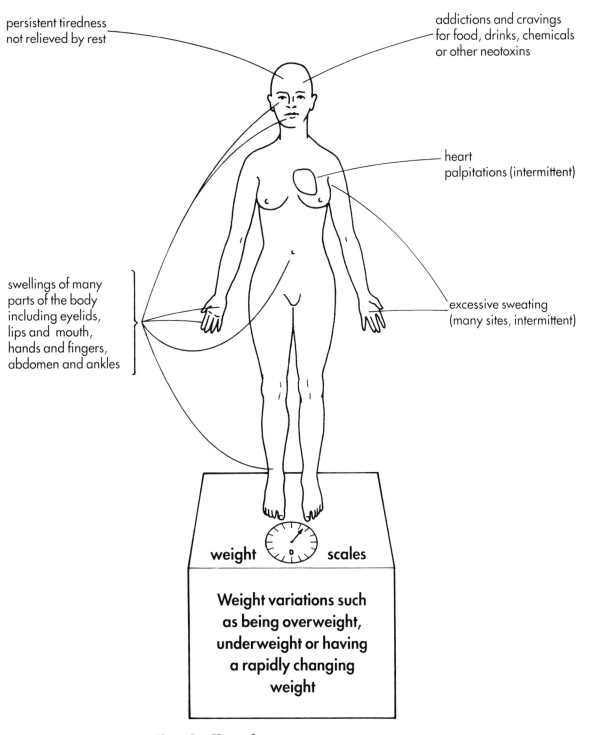

persistent tiredness
not relieved by rest

addictions and cravings
for food, drinks, chemicals
or other neotoxins

heart
palpitations (intermittent)

swellings of many
parts of the body
including eyelids,
lips and mouth,
hands and fingers,
abdomen and ankles

excessive sweating
(many sites, intermittent)

weight   scales

Weight variations such
as being overweight,
underweight or having
a rapidly changing
weight

Figure 1.1 **Generalized allergic symptoms**

GENERALIZED ALLERGIC SYMPTOMS

Symptoms continuous in nature:

● Persistent tiredness that cannot be relieved by rest or sleep. The sufferer wakes up in the morning exhausted. (Other causes must be excluded, anaemia, thyroid disease, cancer); ☐

● Being overweight, underweight, or having a rapidly changing weight. (See height, weight tables in Appendix (Page 235)). ☐

Symptoms usually non-continuous:

● Addiction or intermittent cravings for a food, drink, ☐

chemical or other neotoxin;

● Intermittent swelling of parts of the body (e.g. eyelids, lips, mouth, hands, abdomen and ankles); ☐

● Intermittent palpitations (an irregular and noticeable heartbeat which feels as though there is a small bird fluttering inside your chest); ☐

● Intermittent excessive sweating. ☐

LOCALIZED ALLERGIC SYMPTOMS

Allergy is often localized to one *target organ*. The commonest system affected is the brain followed by those containing smooth muscle, i.e. alimentary tract, lungs, heart and

---

Table 1.3 **Diseases and symptoms of the alimentary canal**

Disease

Disease	Never had disease	Had disease in past	Have disease at present
Anorexia			
COLITIS			
Crohn's disease			
Duodenal ulcer			
Indigestion			
IRRITABLE BOWEL			
OBESITY			
Piles			
Stomach ulcer			
Ulcerative colitis			

Symptom

Symptom	Never had symptom	Had symptom in past	Have symptom at present
ABDOMINAL PAIN			
BLOATING			
COLIC			
CONSTIPATION			
DIARRHOEA			
HUNGER (+++)			
Mouth ulcers			
Nausea			
THIRST (+++)			
Vomiting			
WEIGHT VARIATION			

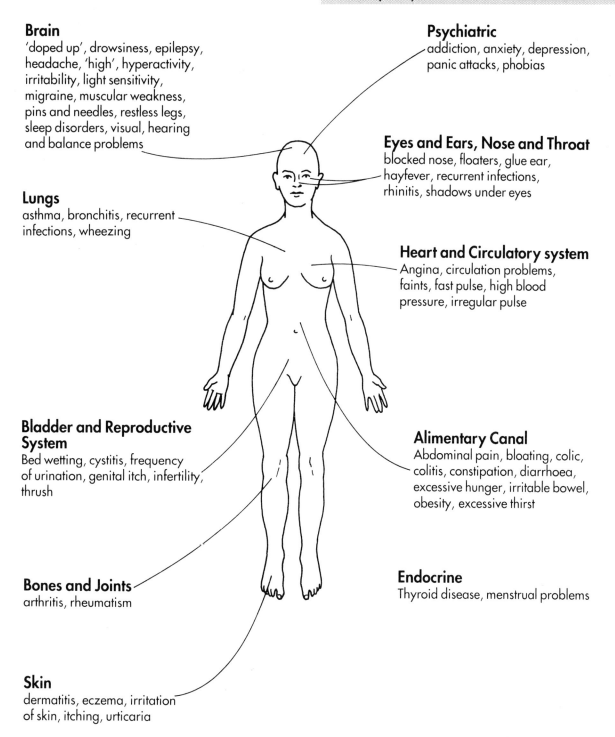

Brain
'doped up', drowsiness, epilepsy, headache, 'high', hyperactivity, irritability, light sensitivity, migraine, muscular weakness, pins and needles, restless legs, sleep disorders, visual, hearing and balance problems

Lungs
asthma, bronchitis, recurrent infections, wheezing

Bladder and Reproductive System
Bed wetting, cystitis, frequency of urination, genital itch, infertility, thrush

Bones and Joints
arthritis, rheumatism

Skin
dermatitis, eczema, irritation of skin, itching, urticaria

Psychiatric
addiction, anxiety, depression, panic attacks, phobias

Eyes and Ears, Nose and Throat
blocked nose, floaters, glue ear, hayfever, recurrent infections, rhinitis, shadows under eyes

Heart and Circulatory system
Angina, circulation problems, faints, fast pulse, high blood pressure, irregular pulse

Alimentary Canal
Abdominal pain, bloating, colic, colitis, constipation, diarrhoea, excessive hunger, irritable bowel, obesity, excessive thirst

Endocrine
Thyroid disease, menstrual problems

Figure 1.2 **Common allergic symptoms and diseases by system**

circulation, and bladder. Other systems, for example bones, joints, glands and skin, are susceptible to a lesser degree.

In this book, a disease or symptom commonly occurring due to failure of the immune and detoxification systems to work properly is given in BLOCK CAPITALS. The diseases and symptoms given in BLOCK CAPITALS are also the easiest ones to cure using the methods outlined in this book. The more symptoms you have from the list, the more likely that they are caused by an allergy. However, if they persist for more than two weeks, or occur intermittently for more than a month, then you should certainly consider allergic causes after your doctor has ruled out other reasons.

Fill in the table below to assess your likelihood of suffering from an allergy.

HOW DO NEOTOXINS CAUSE ALLERGIES?

Neotoxins (e.g. food additives, pesticides) produce allergies by causing a malfunction of the immune and detoxification systems, which then causes secondary damage in other tissues of the body. This damage is initially caused by free radicals, followed by inflammation which causes the release of highly reactive substances such as histamine and prostaglandins. Histamine causes swelling, leakage of fluid from blood vessels and irritation.

There is disagreement among scientists as to how the allergy damages the immune system. Some of the suggested ways include the following:

● **Toxicity**
  This is due to a direct or indirect toxic effect of the neotoxin (e.g. lead, mercury and other heavy metals) on the immune system

---

Table 1.4 **Diseases and symptoms of the lungs, eyes, ears, nose and throat**

Disease

Disease	Never had disease	Had disease in past	Have disease at present
ASTHMA			
Bronchitis			
Conjunctivitis			
GLUE EAR			
HAY FEVER			
RHINITIS			
Sinusitis			

Symptom

Symptom	Never had symptom	Had symptom in past	Have symptom at present
BLOCKED NOSE			
Catarrh			
Cough			
Dry eyes			
FLOATERS			
RECURRENT INFECTIONS			
SHADOWS UNDER EYES			
WHEEZING			

Table 1.5 **Diseases and symptoms of the brain**

Disease

	Never had disease	Had disease in past	Have disease at present
ADDICTION			
Anxiety			
Depression			
Epilepsy			
HYPER-ACTIVITY			
MIGRAINE			
Panic Attacks			
Phobias			
Psychotic illness			
Tinnitus			
Vertigo			

Symptom

	Never had symptom	Had symptom in past	Have symptom at present
'DOPED-UP'			
DROWSINESS			
HEADACHE			
'HIGH'			
IRRITABILITY			
LIGHT SENSITIVITY			
Muscular Weakness			
Pins & Needles			
RECURRENT TIREDNESS			
Restless legs			
Sleep Disorder			
SWEATING			
Visual problems			

Table 1.6 **Diseases and symptoms of the heart and circulatory system**

Disease

	Never had disease	Had disease in past	Have disease at present
Angina			
Circulation Problems			
Heart Attacks			
High Blood Fat			
HIGH BLOOD PRESSURE			

Symptom

	Never had symptom	Had symptom in past	Have symptom at present
FAINTS			
FAST PULSE			
IRREGULAR PULSE			
PALPITATIONS			

Table 1.7 **Diseases and symptoms of the bladder and reproductive system**

Disease

	Never had disease	Had disease in past	Have disease at present
Cystitis			
Frigidity			
Impotence			
Infertility			
Thrush			
Vaginal Discharge			

Symptom

	Never had symptom	Had symptom in past	Have symptom at present
Bed wetting			
Frequency of urination			
Genital itch			

Table 1.8 **Diseases and symptoms of the skin**

Disease

	Never had disease	Had disease in past	Have disease at present
CONTACT DERMATITIS			
ECZEMA			
SKIN IRRITATION			

Symptom

	Never had symptom	Had symptom in past	Have symptom at present
ITCHING			
OEDEMA			
URTICARIA			

and detoxification systems. The detoxification system is overwhelmed by an excessively toxic substance or a less toxic substance in too high an amount.

● **Irritation**
This is due to release of histamine and other highly reactive substances by the neotoxin (e.g. acids and alkalis).

● **Pharmacological**
Many neotoxins (e.g. alcohol, caffeine, nicotine) have a drug-like action on the body. These cause their effects by stimulating 'receptors' on the surface of the cells. These 'receptors' identify specific substances due to the shape of the molecule.

● **Immunological reactions**
The immune system produces antibodies which circulate in the blood. These antibodies cause the release of histamine (e.g. hayfever) and join with foreign proteins to produce immune complexes

Table 1.9 **Diseases and symptoms of the endocrine glands**

Disease

	Never had disease	Had disease in past	Have disease at present
Thyroid Disease			

Symptom

	Never had symptom	Had symptom in past	Have symptom at present
Heavy periods			
Painful periods			

Table 1.10 **Diseases and symptoms of the bones and joints**

Disease

	Never had disease	Had disease in past	Have disease at present
ARTHRITIS			

Symptom

	Never had symptom	Had symptom in past	Have symptom at present
RHEUMATISM			

which can cause activation of the 'complement' system, and white cells which then produce tissue damage (e.g. contact dermatitis).

● **Non-immunological reactions**
This is a very large category and is the cause of a large proportion of allergic problems although the precise mechanism is not known.

● **Intolerance**
This is caused by enzymes not working properly. Enzymes are catalysts produced by the body to assist the biochemical conversion of one substance to another. Enzyme malfunctions can be 'fixed' (non-repairable) or 'non-fixed' (repairable with time).

A 'fixed' enzyme defect is caused by a damaged gene inherited from one or other parent. It will never heal and the possessor of this gene will have an allergic problem throughout life, e.g. coeliac disease, in which the patient cannot eat gluten, a protein present in wheat.

A 'non-fixed' enzyme defect occurs because an enzyme is overused and it becomes 'bruised', for example temporary milk allergy often occurs in infants after a bowel infection. If the enzyme system is 'rested' for a short time (two to six months), then it is usually able to repair itself wholly or partly, and the body goes into a state of 'tolerance'. In this state of 'tolerance' it is possible occasionally (say once a week) to take the neotoxin that previously gave the problem without allergic symptoms.

Table 1.11 **The Weak Link Theory**

Age	Most common allergy	Comments
0–6 months	Loose bowels	
6 mths–2yrs	Eczema	Commoner in boys
2yrs–10yrs	Asthma & Hyperactivity	
10yrs–20yrs	Migraine	
20yrs–30yrs	Colitis	
30yrs–40yrs	Recurrent tiredness, Depression & Premenstrual tension	Commoner in women
40yrs–70yrs	Arthritis	

WHICH FACTORS ARE LIKELY TO MAKE ME ALLERGIC?

There are several recognized factors that increase your risk of suffering from an allergy. One of them is heredity, but this is beyond your control since you cannot choose your parents. Fortunately, however, heredity is much less important than acquired factors, i.e. your environment, which you can control.

The factors that influence an allergy are heredity, age and sex, nutrition, hormonal state, general state of health and total load of neotoxins.

Heredity
This is an allergic tendency (sometimes called atopy) which can be inherited. Your likelihood of being allergic is as follows:

	Likelihood of being allergic
If neither parent is allergic	10–20%
If one parent is allergic	30–50%
If both parents are allergic	40–75%

The factor causing the allergy being inherited is probably a partial or complete enzyme deficiency, giving rise to the allergic symptoms.

Different members of the same family may have different allergic problems at different ages, but the cause is the inherited enzyme defect, revealed by the excess *load of neotoxins* which have overwhelmed the immune and detoxification systems. Any allergic symptom in a member of a family increases the risk of other members of the families suffering from allergy. Your mother has slightly more influence on your risk of allergy than your father. This is because although you inherit an equal number of genes, which form the nucleus of the cell, from both your mother and father, the extra-cellular parts of the cell, e.g. the mitochondria, are inherited exclusively from your mother.

Age and Sex
Allergic disease is more common in young infants and children, especially boys, many allergies *apparently* curing themselves by the age of twenty. Adult women are almost twice as likely to suffer from allergies as men (this is explored in greater depth in Chapter 15).

The age and sex of a patient dictates the particular allergic illness that that person is most likely to suffer from, as described in the *weak link theory* (Table 1.11).

Infants tend to suffer from eczema, older children from asthma, hay fever and hyperactivity. After puberty, and especially childbirth, allergic illnesses become much more common in women e.g. migraine, colitis, recurrent tiredness and arthritis.

If one individual is studied throughout their life, their allergic illnesses will often move from one system to another as they get older, although the underlying allergic susceptibility to a neotoxin (e.g. milk) remains constant.

The weak link theory also explains why an allergy starts or appears in one part of the body but not another. For example, eczema first affects the inner surface of knees and elbows sparing other parts of the body. The reason for this is that skin temperature, humidity, blood supply, exposure to light, non-stretching of the skin on the elbows and knees provide the best conditions for the start of eczema. If the allergy gets worse then eczema may spread over the whole body, but as far as the eczema is concerned the elbows and knees are the weak link.

Nutrition

This is the single most important factor that influences the development of allergy. Its importance starts before birth when the baby is growing in the mother's womb. If the mother does not smoke or drink alcohol, and avoids eating the same few foods (by rotating unpolluted organic foods and drinking spring water), and takes adequate mineral and vitamin intakes, she greatly reduces the likelihood of allergy in her child.

Also, it is important that after birth the baby is *exclusively* breast fed, with no cow's milk bottles at all, and that the mother continues on her unpolluted organic diet and spring water. Neotoxins from polluted food are concentrated into mothers' milk. Ideally, weaning should be postponed until the baby is at least 6 months old. When weaning is started, foods should be rotated (each food taken not more than once every three days).

If the baby has a bowel infection causing diarrhoea (and damage to the bowel wall), all food should be stopped, and the baby should be given spring water only, until the diarrhoea ceases. Despite the extra cost, organic foods are very important for health. They contain the natural balance of proteins, carbohydrates and fats, vitamins and minerals, and should be completely free of chemical contaminants, e.g. colouring, flavourings, E numbers, pesticides, petrochemicals and toxic metals.

Hormonal state

The immune and detoxification systems are influenced by hormones. The level of hormones varies with time of day (circadian rhythm) and, for women, time of the month (menstrual cycle). The time of day at which there is greatest susceptibility to illness is 4.00am. For women the time of the month of greatest susceptibility to illness is the week before their period.

Other habits

Alcohol, smoking and drugs (prescribed or otherwise), all take their toll on the immune system. In addition, sex with many partners increases the risk of infection and consequent neotoxin load. Heterosexual women have an extra problem, in that semen contains high doses of 'foreign' proteins and the substance prostaglandin. Both of these will challenge a woman's immune system.

General state of health

This influences how much resistance a person has to further challenges.

Total load of neotoxins

This is a fundamental concept in Environmental Medicine. The state of your immune

29

system is very strongly influenced by your *total load of neotoxins*. If your food and drink have many additives, and/or you are exposed to many chemicals, and/or electromagnetic radiations, and have a highly stressed lifestyle, then you are more likely to suffer an allergic problem. *The higher the total load, the greater the risk of allergy.*

WHAT ARE THE COMMON CAUSES OF NEOTOXINS?

Biological neotoxins

These have increased geometrically since the Second World War, when intensive farming methods started in earnest. Food poisoning (an infection), is now depressingly common, and most non-organic meat contains hormones, antibiotics and food additives. Water supplies are treated with chemicals, and contain pesticides and heavy metals.

Chemicals

One hundred years ago there were approximately 150 chemicals in common use. Now there are 60,000. The consumer society has flooded the world with petrochemical fumes and pesticides residues. In addition, organic chemists have succeeded in producing chemicals (halocarbons) that are much more dangerous because of the carbon-chlorine bond they contain. These halocarbons appear to cause much more damage to the immune system, and sources include PCBs from electrical devices, organochlorine, pesticides, cleaning solvents and CFCs in refrigerators and aerosols.

Physical

One hundred years ago there were no household electrical devices, and consequently, very few synthetic electric and magnetic fields. In the western world it is now impossible to find a control population which does not live in an 'electric smog' created by heating and lighting circuits, especially caused by motors and transformers.

Mental

A high level of mental stress is now the expected norm for city-dwellers. Mental stress contributes to the total load of neotoxins and makes the body more susceptible to an allergy.

WHAT DETERMINES IF I WILL SUFFER FROM A NEOTOXIN?

The factors that decide whether you will suffer from a neotoxin are:

- The *total load of neotoxins* (biological, chemical, physical and mental);
- Individual susceptibility. This is determined by two factors:
  a) the set of genes you inherit from your parents;
  b) general state of health.

The inherited portion of your individual susceptibility cannot be changed, however, the acquired portion is dependent on your environment, and you can change it to such an extent as to cancel out most genetic defects. The genes you inherit will decide whether you have any defective enzymes. These defective enzymes can cause disease which may be revealed by environmental challenges. Scientists have already found the defective gene that causes asthma and cystic fibrosis.

The dose of neotoxins received by a person can be worked out by using the formula:

Dose of = Amount of × 'Proximity' to × Time
neotoxin neotoxin source of exposed
neotoxin to neotoxin

However, the dose is not the same as the biological effect, which can be worked out by using the formula:

$$\text{Biological effect} = \begin{array}{c}\text{Dose of}\\\text{neotoxin}\end{array} \times \begin{array}{c}\text{Individual}\\\text{susceptibility}\\\text{to neotoxin}\end{array}$$

and

$$\begin{array}{c}\text{Individual}\\\text{Susceptibility}\end{array} = \begin{array}{c}\text{Genetic}\\\text{influences}\end{array} \times \begin{array}{c}\text{Acquired}\\\text{environmental}\\\text{influences}\end{array}$$

The way to beat allergies is explained more fully in Chapter 6, but there are three basic rules:

- Reduce your total load of neotoxins;
- Reduce the neotoxin(s) to which you are particularly susceptible;
- Use sleep, rest, exercise, vitamin and mineral supplements to get yourself back to positive health.

WHAT'S WRONG WITH CONVENTIONAL MEDICINE'S WAY OF TREATING ALLERGIES?

Conventional medicine treats allergic disease by giving tablets, (antihistamines), and creams, (steroids), that *suppress* the symptoms.

This is basically a flawed approach to treatment. The best way to treat allergies is not just to treat the symptom(s) but to remove the cause, i.e. the neotoxin.

The symptoms caused by the neotoxin are often the body's attempt to heal itself. For example, diarrhoea is the body's attempt to flush out the offending substance from the bowel. In the same way, the runny nose of hayfever is trying to flush out pollen from the nostrils. To suppress these compensatory mechanisms is merely directing the problem into another system. For example, when topical steroid creams are used to treat eczema, the skin eruption disappears but the problem is transferred to the lungs and increases the likelihood of asthma.

WHY CAN'T I ACCURATELY DESCRIBE THE SYMPTOMS OF MY ALLERGY TO MY DOCTOR?

A large proportion of patients attending their general practitioner, are unable to define their problem precisely. They complain of vague

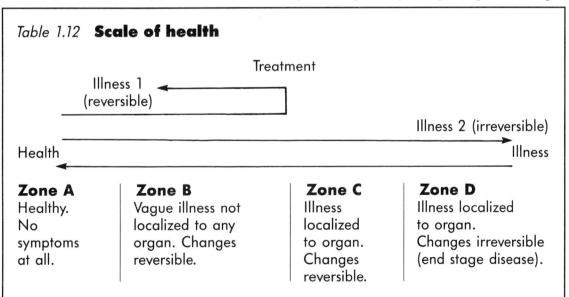

Table 1.12 **Scale of health**

Zone A	Zone B	Zone C	Zone D
Healthy. No symptoms at all.	Vague illness not localized to any organ. Changes reversible.	Illness localized to organ. Changes reversible.	Illness localized to organ. Changes irreversible (end stage disease).

symptoms with descriptions of 'feeling off', 'under the weather', 'tired all the time and having no energy'.

To understand the reason for this, it is helpful to look at the several stages that any disease goes through as shown in the Scale of Health overleaf.

Table 1.12 gives the range of health/illness, from complete health at the left-hand side of the diagram, to complete illness, at the right-hand side of the diagram. In the first stage of disease (Zone B), the body is exposed to a neotoxin, e.g. a virus, and the illness produced is vague and cannot be localized to any one organ. At this stage the disease is still reversible. If the neotoxin exposure continues, the illness becomes localized to a system, e.g. a temporary pain in the joint, but is still reversible (stage C). If no further steps are taken to modify and improve the lifestyle, then the illness becomes irreversible, (Zone D), causing permanent arthritis. The ideal time to act is when the disease is in Zone B or Zone C, when the allergy is still reversible and a full recovery is possible (as in illness 1 above). In comparison, treatment of irreversible disease in Zone D (end-stage disease) is difficult, and perfect results cannot normally be obtained (as in illness 2 above).

Sometimes patients with allergic symptoms are found to have normal blood tests. In spite of obvious suffering, their doctors insist that the patients are not ill. Unfortunately these doctors are not treating the patients but the blood tests, which are not yet sophisticated enough to show allergic disease.

WHAT SETS OFF ALLERGIES? (the Trigger Event)

Many diseases, including allergic ones, often occur following a *trigger event*, such as an accident, bereavement, infection or massive

exposure to a neotoxin. Once the illness has started, there is often a permanent change, and the illness continues even if the trigger event is then removed.

The reason that an illness occurs after a trigger event is due to a hidden weakness. This weakness only becomes evident after a trigger event reveals the problem. To use the analogy of a large boulder sitting on the edge of a cliff, compared to another boulder some distance from the edge along the plain (see below). The first boulder 'A' requires a relatively small push to get it to fall to the valley below. However, the second boulder 'B' on the plain is in a much safer position, and has to be pushed a long way across the plain before it will fall off the edge of the cliff.

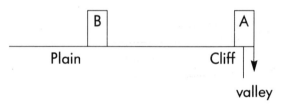

The way that an allergic illness starts is similar to the boulder analogy. People who have a hidden weakness to a neotoxin, (like Boulder 'A') require a relatively small push or trigger event to precipitate their allergic disease. Other people without this hidden weakness have considerably more resistance to a trigger event, but if you expose anyone to a powerful enough trigger event, e.g. the explosion at Bhopal, then they will become ill.

WHAT ARE THE STAGES OF AN ALLERGIC RESPONSE?

The stages of an allergic response are now understood, thanks to the original pioneering work of Professor Selye together with clinical observation by Dr Theron Randolph and Dr Richard Mackarness. The description that

Stages

follows is the *general adaption syndrome*, which is of particular significance in the explanation of allergies.

1. When a neotoxin is first taken it produces an immediate 'alarm' reaction (see Figure 1.3). In this alarm reaction the subject feels unwell, but if no further neotoxin is taken there will be a recovery to the normal baseline (Stage A).

2. If, however, the neotoxin, e.g. cigarette or alcohol, is taken constantly (Stage B), after a brief 'alarm' phase the subject progresses to a state where he actually feels 'pepped up' and better than usual. This elated feeling is due to the neotoxin 'masking' the allergy. This stage is known as 'resistance' or 'adaption' because even though the neotoxin is harming the subject, he is able to cope with it and even feels well because the immune and detoxification systems are working overtime to manage.

3. If the neotoxin is removed for more than about 12 hours, a withdrawal reaction will occur which feels like a 'hangover'. The subject identifies this hangover as his or her allergy. If, however, the neotoxin is taken every day, (or at least every three days, since it takes about that time to clear an edible neotoxin from the body) a withdrawal hangover is prevented.

4. If the neotoxin is removed for more than three days, then after the hangover, which lasts for about three further days, the subject will start to feel better (Stage C). If, after 5 days of abstinence, the 'adaption' phase is lost and the subject is re-exposed to the neotoxin, the alarm reaction will immediately recur.

5. Eventually, after a long period, if the neotoxin has been taken continually, (or at least every three days), the 'masked' allergy stage will pass and be replaced by the exhaustion stage (Stage D). In this exhaustion stage each new exposure to the neotoxin will no longer give a 'lift', but an immediate bad reaction.

WHY DON'T I KNOW TO WHICH NEOTOXIN I AM ALLERGIC?

There are two major reasons why you don't know to which neotoxin you are allergic. There are two facets of masking:

● First, you don't improve initially when you stop exposing yourself to the neotoxin that is giving you the allergy. In fact, paradoxically, you will often initially get *worse* due to a withdrawal reaction which feels like a hangover. You usually won't start to feel fully well for three to six days,

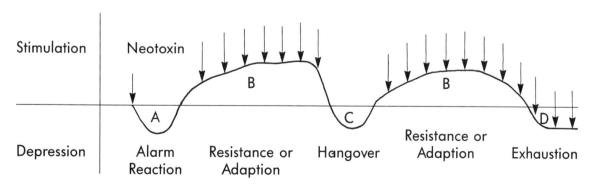

Figure 1.3 **The general adaption syndrome**

by which time your body has removed a large proportion of the neotoxin(s).

- Second, there is a delay between challenging yourself with a neotoxin and a reaction occurring, and in many cases there is no reaction or else the neotoxin actually makes you feel better. The delay may be up to 24 or 48 hours. However, after the elimination process you will react more severely and faster to the neotoxin, (this is a state called hypersensitivity, which will persist for up to several months until you gain a tolerance to the neotoxin).

Consequently, you don't know which neotoxin(s) you are allergic to because you don't get better when you remove it (and may even get worse), and you don't get worse straight away after reintroducing it back into your life. Allergic disease is often missed because patients in Stage B with masked allergy feel in positive good health provided that they get their daily fix of neotoxin(s), e.g. coffee, chocolate. They feel quite sure that their neotoxin makes them feel well and probably do not consult a doctor until they go on to Stage C or D.

WHAT AFFECTS THE SPEED OF REACTION FOLLOWING EXPOSURE TO A NEOTOXIN?

The body may react very quickly or rather slowly following exposure to a neotoxin. A true anaphylactic reaction (which is relatively rare), can occur within seconds of exposure and is usually associated with tingling around the mouth, swelling of the lips and tongue, and possibly even life-threatening drop in blood pressure and swelling around the air tubes. Excluding anaphylactic reactions, most other allergic reactions occur after exposure with a delay of between half an hour and two days, with an upper limit of 72 hours. The factors that govern the time taken for the body to react to the neotoxin are:

- General health of the patient, and the allergic state of the patient (whether in a state of tolerance, hypersensitivity or masked allergy);
- The distance that the neotoxin has to travel through the body. Neotoxins acting on the nose immediately arrive at their target organ. Equally, food starts to produce allergic symptoms in the upper alimentary canal as soon as it is eaten. If a food has to be transported in the blood to a more distant target organ, such as the lungs, then here is usually a longer delay before the food induced asthma starts. Before allergy can start in a distant target organ the food has to be absorbed, passed through the liver and then transported by the blood stream to that organ. The allergic symptoms that usually take the longest to show themselves are those in skin and joints, since there is quite a delay before food reaches these targets.

SUMMARY

- Allergies are very common and occur at any time after the first exposure to a neotoxin (poison of the twentieth century).
- The four sources of neotoxins are biological, chemical, physical and mental.
- Allergies occur because a neotoxin(s) stops the immune and detoxification systems from working properly.

- Allergies can cause a very wide variety of symptoms and diseases. The symptoms and diseases produced in any specific individual depends upon the weak link in their body, and this weak link will vary with age.
- The important general symptoms of allergy include, permanent tiredness unrelieved by rest, incorrect weight for height or rapidly changing body weight, addictions, intermittent body swellings, sweating and palpitations.
- Allergic illnesses include asthma, hayfever, eczema, urticaria, arthritis, irritable bowel syndrome, migraine, depression and anxiety.
- A tendency to allergy is often inherited but can also be caused by an unhealthy lifestyle, or a trigger event.
- The way to heal allergies is to:
  i) Reduce your total load of neotoxins;
  ii) Reduce the neotoxin(s) to which you are particularly susceptible.
  iii) Use sleep, rest, exercise, vitamin and mineral supplements to get yourself back to positive health.

CHAPTER TWO

FOODS, WATER, INFECTIONS AND YOUR HEALTH

An alien from outer space would be forgiven for thinking that the food industry's secret plan was to wage biological warfare on the population of the world. The increasing adulteration of food and drink with additives, hormones, antibiotics and many chemicals, together with the presence of food-borne infections, means that most people are digging a grave with their own teeth, and the vast rise in allergies is completely understandable – even to be expected.

The biological neotoxins that cause allergies are contained in:

● **Food**
This includes all edible matter and also all substances *deliberately* added to food, e.g. hormones, antibiotics, colouring, flavourings, preservatives, antioxidants, emulsifiers, stabilizers, sweeteners, minerals, hydrocarbons, modified starches, acids, anti-caking agents, anti-foaming agents, bases, buffers, bulking agents, firming agents, flavour modifiers, flour-bleaching agents, flour improvers, glazing agents, humectants, liquid freezants, packaging, gases, propellants, releasing agents, sequestrants and solvents.

Although they will be mentioned in this chapter all *food contaminants* (i.e. things that have found their way into food by accident)

will be dealt with in depth in Chapter 3.
● **Water**
Water is greatly under-estimated as a source of allergy. Despite reassurances to the contrary, an increasing number of people cannot drink tap water without becoming ill. Tap water is routinely treated with chlorine, aluminium salts and fluorides, all of which may cause disease. All water contaminants, (i.e. things that have found their way into the water by accident, e.g. pesticides, trichlorethylene, PCBs), will be dealt with in Chapter 3.

● **Infections**
Infections can be caused by bacteria, viruses, fungi or parasites. This book deals with environmentally-induced diseases and, consequently, this chapter will look at infections from the following sources:
   a) infections present in food
   b) infections present in water
   c) infections caused by occupations

● **Animals**
Animal hair and fur cause allergic conditions of the eye, ear, nose, throat and lungs. Certain insects, typically the house dust mite, may cause similar problems.

● **Plants**
Pollens from trees, bushes and plants can cause allergic conditions of eyes, ears, nose, throat and lungs. This allergy is called

hayfever. Fungal spores may cause similar problems.

FOOD

You are what you eat

The real truth behind this well-known statement is brought home when you appreciate that the body completely replaces every molecule with a new similar one every 7 to 10 years. Therefore, if you eat food heavily polluted with neotoxins your body will become full of them, (bioaccumulation) and, consequently, you will stand a very high chance of suffering from allergic symptoms and diseases.

Why does food allergy occur?

There are several proposed explanations, but one of the most widely accepted is that food allergy is caused by a *failure of the body to adapt to the change in the diet since the Stone Age*. To put it another way, we are giving our bodies the wrong food, so they do not work properly. It is like putting diesel fuel in a petrol engine.

The human body was 'designed' to digest and live on the Stone-Age diet. The essence of the Stone-Age diet was *variety*, and an absence of neotoxins. Stone Age people would eat everything that they could find that wasn't poisonous. This would include all sections of a plant, starting from the roots at the bottom to the buds at the top, taking in stems, leaves, fruits, berries and nuts on the way. Equally, all non-poisonous animals were eaten, and not just a small variety of large mammals, chickens and relatively few species of fish as are eaten in the late twentieth century. Instead, mammals both large and small were eaten, together with a wide variety of birds, reptiles and fish. Stone Age humans not only ate the above animals, which are all vertebrates, but would also eat a very wide variety of invertebrates, including molluscs, crustaceans, insects and worms.

Since the Stone Age there have been three major changes in the diet:

- About 10,000 years ago, Stone Age people ceased being nomads and settled down in one place, cultivating wheat and cereals, and keeping hens and cattle. Dairy products, wheat products and eggs were then eaten daily.
- Several hundred years ago, sailing ships became faster and were used to import large quantities of common allergic foods like citrus fruits, tea, coffee, cocoa, sugar which were then available all the year round. Before this time, any fruit would be available for only three months of the year, since it could not be stored for long in the absence of refrigeration. After the three months of availability the food was compulsively removed from the diet for the following nine months until the next season came around.
- Since World War Two, the food industry has hugely increased its output by battery cultivation of animals, wide use of insecticides and fertilizers, and petrochemical additives (E numbers). These petrochemical additives are now so widely used that it is difficult to have a diet completely free of colours, preservatives, antioxidants, emulsifiers and stabilizers.

As well as being chemically polluted, modern production methods yield food that looks attractive but contains abnormal amounts of vitamins, minerals, proteins, carbohydrates and fats. Since the food has been 'forced', made to grow rapidly, it has much less vitality and health-giving properties than organic food. Some oranges grown in California under intensive farming conditions have been found to contain no Vitamin C at all!

37

An increasing number of people cannot eat the modern diet, which is repetitive, lacking in variety, and gives high daily levels of the following: milk, cheese, butter, eggs, beef, wheat, wheat products, tea, coffee, cocoa, sugar, citrus fruits and additives. These particular foods are the most common cause of food allergy, especially the very high daily load of refined carbohydrates such as white flour and sugar, which would have been almost completely absent from the Stone Age diet. The body cannot cope with an excessive amount or repetition of any one food, and protests by exhibiting allergic symptoms and diseases.

Which food is most likely to cause an allergy?

Any food that is taken repeatedly may cause an allergy, although some foods are highly allergic and are more likely to cause problems than others (see table below). Cooking tends to reduce the likelihood of allergy, since it 'fixes' large protein molecules, breaking them down into smaller molecules which are less likely to induce an immune response and are more easily processed by the detoxification system.

However, the substances most likely to cause allergy are fat soluble (e.g. pesticides), and easily penetrate the blood/brain barrier to get into the brain. They also remain in the body for a very long time (10 to 20 years), since they are firmly bound to the fat stores. Since the average adult eats and drinks a tonne of food each year, containing approximately 6lbs of food additives, even a small amount of pollution in a meal becomes a large amount when viewed cumulatively.

What are food additives?

These are chemicals added to food to 'improve' the colour, flavour, shelf-life and marketability of the food products. Before World War Two relatively few food additives were used, but in the western world it is now very difficult to get a diet that is completely free of additives. The best way is to eat only fresh organic food and nothing from a packet or tin.

What are the categories of food additives?

Food additives are usually given an 'E' number (designated by a European committee) which denotes which category of substance the additive falls into:

Permitted colours (E100–E180)
Preservatives (E200–E290)
Permitted Antioxidants (E300–E321)
Emulsifiers and Stabilizers (occasional numbers (E322 and E494)
Sweeteners (E420–E421)
Mineral Hydrocarbons (E905–E907)
Modified Starches (E1400–E1442)

Other additives include acids, anti-caking agents, anti-foaming agents, bases, buffers, bulking agents, firming agents, flavour modifiers, flour-bleaching agents, flour-improvers, glazing agents, humectants, liquid freezants, packaging gases, propellants, release agents, sequestrants and solvents.

What are the E numbers for flavourings?

There are *several thousand* different flavourings, and consequently they have no 'E' numbers.

What are the sources of food additives?

Some food additives come from natural sources, e.g. chlorophyll, and are possibly safe. Others are the products of the petrochemical industry and practitioners of Environmental Medicine recognize that they give rise to food allergies, especially in children. However,

Table 2.1 **Foods which are most likely to cause an allergy**

Highly allergic	Moderately allergic	Slightly allergic
Additives	Apples	Apricots
Antibiotics (fed to animals)	Avocados	Artichokes
	Bananas	Asparagus
Alcoholic drinks	Beef	Broccoli
Azo dyes	Berries	Carrots
Bacon	Buckwheat	Chard
Barley	Cabbage	Cranberries
Beans	Cauliflower	Figs
Butter	Celery	Grapes
Cheese	Cherries	Honey
Chocolate	Chicken	Lettuce
Citrus fruits	Coconut	Marrow
Cocoa	Cucumber	Peaches
Coffee	Egg yolk	Pears
Cola drinks	Fish	Raisins
Corn	Frozen foods (frequent additives)	Rice
Egg (White)		Rye
Ham	Garlic	Sugar (maple, sorghum)
Legumes	Green & red peppers	Sweet potatoes
Milk	Lamb	Tapioca
Milk products	Mangos	Turkey
Mustard	Melons	
Oats	Mint	
Onions & leeks	Mushrooms	
Peanuts	Nuts	
Peas	Plums	
Pineapple	Potatoes	
Pork	Prunes	
Sausages	Root vegetables	
Soya bean products	Safflower	
Sugars (beet, cane, corn, molasses)	Shellfish	
Tea	Spices	
Tinned foods	Spinach	
Tomatoes	String beans	
Vinegar		
Wheat (especially white)		
Wine (especially red)		
Yeast		
Yoghurt		

merely because a food additive is from a 'natural' source does not mean that it is safe; e.g. annatto [160(b)] comes from the tropical annatto tree, but causes a reaction in many people.

How do food additives cause harm?

This mechanism is at present poorly understood, but it would appear that food additives disrupt the detoxification system by interfering with enzyme systems in the liver and cells, depleting the body's stores of essential vitamins, and trace metals like zinc.

Which additives should be avoided by children?

Ideally, children should eat only fresh food, without any additives at all. However, the following food additives are known to be capable of causing hyperactivity in children, and should be completely avoided by children under 16 years and by expectant mothers:

E102	Tartrazine
E104	Quinoline Yellow
107	Yellow 2G
E110	Sunset Yellow FCF
E120	Cochineal
E122	Carmoisine
E123	Amaranth
E124	Ponceau 4R
E127	Erythrosine
128	Red 2G
E132	Indigo Carmine
E133	Brilliant Red FCF
E150	Caramel
E151	Black PN
154	Brown FK
155	Brown HT
E1606	Annatlo
E210	Benzoic Acid
E211	Sodium Benzoate
E220	Sulphur Dioxide
E250	Sodium Nitrate
E251	Potassium Nitrate
E320	Butylated Hydroxyanisole
E321	Butylated Hydroxytoluene

The following additives should be avoided by asthmatics, aspirin-sensitive people, infants, young children and hyperactive children:

E212	Potassium Benzoate
E213	Calcium Benzoate
E214	Ethyl 4-hydroxybenzoate
E215	Ethyl 4-hydroxybenzoate, sodium salt
E216	Propyl 4-hydroxybenzoate
E217	Propyl 4-hydroxybenzoate, sodium salt
E218	Methyl 4-hydroxybenzoate
E219	Methyl 4-hydroxybenzoate, sodium salt
E310	Propyl gallate
E311	Octyl gallate
E312	Dodecyl gallate
621	Monosodium glutamate
622	Monopotassium glutamate
623	Calcium glutamate
627	Guanosine 5-(disodium phosphate)
631	Inosine 5-(disodium phosphate)
635	Sodium 5-ribonucleotide

(Some special numbers do not have an 'E' prefix because they have not yet been fully evaluated by the European community.)

How much additive does it require to make me ill?

Some patients are highly susceptible to food additives, and as little as one tenth of a teaspoonful of an additive-containing food may be enough to set off a reaction. Tartrazine (E102) is one of the most toxic additives, and a susceptible patient can sustain a severe allergic reaction after eating only a few micrograms (enough to cover the sharp end of a pin!).

How long does it take for a reaction to occur with a food additive?

A reaction may occur within seconds, but often will not show itself for 24 hours, with an outside limit of 72 hours. As a general rule, the more severe the reaction, the quicker it appears. You may feel better after eating a food additive because your allergy is said to be 'masked'. If you remove the additive from your diet for more than 2 to 3 days, then a withdrawal reaction that feels like a hangover will probably occur.

How long does a food allergy last with a food additive?

The food allergy lasts for as long as it takes the body to completely clear itself of the additive. This usually takes about 3–5 days.

How can I tell if there is an additive in my food?

Look at the label! (See example below.) Manufacturers are obliged by law to list all ingredients in their products in descending order of weight. There are several exceptions, including 'take away' foods, individually wrapped sweets, unwrapped foods, alcoholic drinks with more than 1.2% alcohol content, and medicines.

Be very careful to read the food labels completely literally. A food whose label states 'free of artificial colouring' may contain 'natural' colouring, flavour, antioxidants and many other additives. Also make sure that you continue to read labels even for familiar products, since manufacturers sometimes substitute ingredients due to supply-shortages or changes in the price of ingredients.

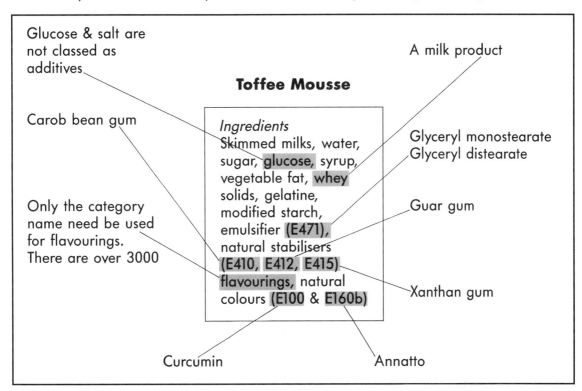

Glucose & salt are not classed as additives

A milk product

Toffee Mousse

Carob bean gum

Ingredients
Skimmed milks, water, sugar, glucose, syrup, vegetable fat, whey solids, gelatine, modified starch, emulsifier (E471), natural stabilisers (E410, E412, E415) flavourings, natural colours (E100 & E160b)

Glyceryl monostearate
Glyceryl distearate

Guar gum

Only the category name need be used for flavourings. There are over 3000

Xanthan gum

Curcumin

Annatto

Unfortunately, reading the label is only useful up to a point. Sometimes manufacturers are vague about an ingredient, for example 'vegetable oil' could mean wheat oil, corn oil, soya oil, peanut oil or sunflower oil. An allergic patient might react to one of these oils but not to another, but has no way of knowing which one is contained in the food.

There is also the problem of 'hidden additives'. Many foods are made from ingredients that have already been processed themselves. For example, the main ingredient of cake is 'flour'. However, it is not possible to tell from the description 'flour' whether there are any additives, such as bleaching agents, raising agents or colourings. A person allergic to 'flour' may not be reacting to the flour itself but to the unlabelled additives. Cake consists mostly of flour, so an additive put in during the flour processing can be present at a high level in the cake, without warning.

How do you diagnose food allergy?

There are five stages to diagnosing food allergy.

Suspicion

You should suspect food allergy if you have any of the symptoms or diseases listed in Chapter 1 (page 22). Allergy is greatly underdiagnosed. You can't find an allergy if you don't suspect it in the first place. Discovery depends upon the prepared mind.

Pre-testing and recording of diet and symptoms

Fill in a diet diary (see p. 43) for a week, writing down *everything* that you eat and drink, including snacks. Score your symptoms immediately *before* each meal, using the rating system shown at the bottom of the diet diary.

Discuss the food allergy testing with your doctor. The testing works best if you are not taking any medication at all, even vitamins and minerals. However, you must not stop prescribed tablets without the specific advice of your doctor. Medicines often contain additives, such as colourings and flavourings, and the bulk of the tablet is not active ingredient but compacted milk sugar (lactose), or cornflour. If you are allergic to prescribed drugs which you continue taking, then the symptoms will not disappear on the exclusion diet.

Weigh yourself naked first thing in the morning, (after emptying your bladder, and if possible after opening your bowels), and last thing at night.

Use the method of pulse testing. Take your pulse immediately before meals and count it for 60 seconds. Make sure you have been sitting still for 2 minutes before testing, and have not exerted yourself violently in the previous 5 minutes. After the meal take your pulse after 20 minutes, 1 hour and 2 hours, writing down the rate on the diet diary in the column marked 'Pulse Rate'. If your pulse rate goes up or down more than 20 beats a minute after a meal, then you should suspect that you have just eaten a food to which you are allergic.

It may seem surprising that the pulse rate can become faster *or* slower with an allergic reaction, but this is a common effect found in most organs. If a system (e.g. bowels), is undergoing an allergic reaction, it may be stimulated (diarrhoea) or suppressed (constipation), but in either case it does not work in the usual fashion. The reaction caused in the body is usually dose-dependent. A small dose of neotoxin causes stimulation but a larger dose causes suppression. The pulse test is the most accurate indicator of allergy during the elimination diet and challenge stages.

When you have recorded your meals, pulse rate and symptoms, it may emerge that a

Table 2.2 **Diet Diary**

Name: .... Date: ....   Weight (Naked) am ....
Food challenge ....   pm ....
(for challenge stage only)

Time	Food	Drink	Pulse Rate (bpm)	Symptoms 0–4	Comments
Breakfast					
Mid-morning					
Lunch					
Mid-afternoon					
Tea					
Supper					

Instructions: Count your pulse for 1 minute before your meal, then 20 mins, 1 hr & 2 hrs after meal. Write down the score in beats per minute in 'pulse rate column'. Score your symptoms *before* each meal – use the scoring system.

0 = no symptoms   3 = severe symptoms
1 = mild symptoms   4 = very severe symptoms
2 = moderate symptoms

particular food or drink makes you ill. You can avoid this food or drink when you start on the elimination diet.

Excluding for Allergic Foods

This can be carried out in two ways:

1. **The 5-day fast.** This involves eating no food at all for 5 days. The only thing taken is bottled spring water. However, most people in the western world are not used to fasting, and the 5-day fast should not be carried out without the assistance of another responsible person. Ideally, it should be carried out under the supervision of a practitioner in Environmental Medicine possibly in a specially equipped hospital ward.

2. **The exclusion diet.** This is a more practical proposition for people who are at work or with family commitments. An exclusion diet means coming off _all_ the foods to which you are likely to be allergic for 7–10 days.

    Most food-allergic people react to more than one food. If you are allergic to four foods, your exclusion diet can be compared to a door with four bolts on it: you won't be able to open the door until _all_ the bolts are drawn back. Similarly, you won't recover fully until _all_ the allergic foods are removed from your diet.

    On the day you start the exclusion diet it is a good idea to clear your bowel by taking the mild laxative Epsom Salts (magnesium sulphate). This will clear the bowel of food that you ate the day before you started the exclusion diet. You should take two teaspoonfuls of the Epsom Salts dissolved in half a pint of warm spring water. Smokers should make every effort to give up, or at least reduce their consumption to the minimum, since

smoking is a massive cause of internal pollution, and makes most allergies worse.

Drink plenty of pure spring water from glass bottles as this will help to flush out the neotoxins. Spring water in plastic bottles should not be taken, as chemicals from the plastic leach into the spring water.

Take plenty of exercise and arrange to take saunas while on the exclusion diet. The body excretes the neotoxin through sweat, which is produced during exercise and saunas. There is no calorie restriction on the diet and there is no need for you to feel hungry. In spite of this, you are likely to lose weight, because a lot of retained water is lost as the allergy disappears.

Plan your meals in advance and buy only organic foods which are clear of chemicals and additives. Don't eat any processed food (i.e., anything in a packet or tin). If in doubt about a food or a food source, then leave it out. Be sure to read all the labels very carefully, since there are many 'hidden' foods (see page 51). Highly allergic foods like milk, wheat or eggs are used in the preparation of a wide range of common foods. Unfortunately, these foods are often not clearly labelled, and you may unwittingly find yourself eating something that is not permitted in your exclusion diet.

Self-catering is essential, because only then do you know precisely what you are eating. Don't eat in restaurants, because you have no control over the ingredients used. Don't start an exclusion diet during a holiday period like Christmas, when dietary restrictions will prove difficult. You should use bottled water for drinking, washing food, cooking and brushing your teeth. When cooking, use steel or glass cooking utensils; don't use teflon non-stick pans, aluminium or plastic. Don't eat food that has been wrapped in plastic. Don't use toothpaste; use bottled water on its own instead. Don't chew gum or take mints or non-prescribed medicines.

It is essential to keep up your diet diary. Continue to take your pulse before and after meals and weigh yourself in the morning and evening.

It is usual for you to feel worse for the first 3–4 days of the exclusion diet. This is the withdrawal reaction and feels like a hangover. You are particularly likely to crave foods to which you are allergic. ✗ However, you mustn't give up, since taking even a small amount of a food to which you are allergic invalidates the exclusion diet and you will have to start again. Remember that 95 per cent compliance to the diet doesn't give 95 per cent improvement.

The common symptoms that you are likely to experience during the hangover period are: *first 1–4 days*

- a severe headache;
- a 'flu-like' illness with no temperature;
- marked irritability;
- feeling as though you are 'walking through treacle';
- feeling as though you are floating.

Fortunately, these symptoms rapidly pass, and then on days 5–9, provided that you have removed the appropriate foods, you should start to feel clear-headed, with lots of energy and 'get up and go'.

While you are on the exclusion diet it is also important to reduce your *total load* of other neotoxins, i.e., chemicals, radiation and stress. (Chapters, 3, 4 and 5 respectively give you details of these dangers.)

Deciding which exclusion diet you should take is a difficult matter. Ideally it should be selected by a practitioner of Environmental Medicine. The best exclusion diet for you will depend on your whole symptom picture. Part II has a chapter on each of the major allergic diseases and there are appropriate exclusion diets in each chapter.

There are two types of general exclusion diets which help a wide variety of allergic illnesses. The first is the Stone Age diet, which is the diet that humans have lived on for about nine-tenths of their existence. The second is called the Oligoantigenic diet (oligo = few), and this is made up of the few foods that are unlikely to cause food allergies.

The Stone Age diet

This is an approximation to the largely carnivorous diet eaten by humans more than 10,000 years ago. It is cereal-free, dairy-free and chemical-free. One of the main reasons for the success of the Stone Age diet is that it does not overload the body with large amounts of carbohydrates which are the mainstay of the late twentieth century diet. The human body seems to be able to deal with high protein and high fat intake, but not a high carbohydrate intake.

When eating the Stone Age diet, it is important for you to take a wide variety of the allowed foods. Don't just stick to meat and two vegetables. Providing that you eat a *wide* variety of the allowed foods then you can stay on the Stone Age diet indefinitely (as Stone Age humans did).

The Stone Age Diet
Allowed

Fresh meats (organic if possible):
  beef, free range chicken, duck, goose, hare, partridge, pheasant, pigeon, pork, rabbit, turkey, venison.

Fish
  all kinds especially round fish (like cod) rather than flat fish (like plaice).

Fruit & vegetables
> organic without sprays or chemicals. Peel or wash in spring water before cooking in spring water.

Drinks:
> spring water in glass bottles

Seasoning:
> salt

Oils and margarines:
> sunflower and olive oil

Nuts:
> all kinds

Pulses:
> all kinds

Completely avoid
Cereals:
> barley, bread and biscuits, corn, millet, oats, rice, wheat and all wheat products (see hidden foods page 51)

Milk products:
> all milk products – butter, cheese, cream and yoghurt (see hidden foods page 51)

Eggs:
> (see hidden foods page 51)

Sugars:
> chocolate and sweets, soft drinks, white and brown sugar

Processed foods:
> tinned meat and fish, crisps, processed nuts, bacon, smoked fish, kippers

Drinks:
> alcohol, coffee, tea

Chemicals:
> any packaged or processed food that contains chemicals

The Oligoantigenic Diet

These are selected from foods that are less likely to cause allergies. If, however, you know yourself to be allergic to a food in the sample diets below, substitute another food from the 'slightly allergic foods' given on page 39. Dairy products, berries and nuts, pulses (legumes), and highly allergic cereals have been avoided. Take food from organic sources wherever possible.

Sample oligoantigenic diets
Allowed

Diet 1
Meat	Duck
Starch	Rice and rice flour
Oils	Sunflower oil
Fruit	Grapes and grape juice
Vegetables	Carrots, parsnips and swedes
Other	Asparagus and apricots

Diet 2
Meat	Rabbit
Starch	Potato and potato flour
Oils	Olive oil
Fruit	Peeled pears and pear juice
Vegetables	Broccoli, cauliflower, cabbage and sprouts
Other	Marrow and rhubarb

Pip and nut free diet
Completely avoid

Berries	blackberries, loganberries, raspberries, strawberries
Gooseberry	blackcurrants, currants, gooseberries, redcurrant, whitecurrant
Plum	almonds, apricots, cherries, nectarines, peaches, plums, prunes, sloes
Grape	grapes, raisins, sultanas, tartar, wine/alcohol

Pomes	apples, cider (vinegar), pears, quinces, rosehips
Citrus & citrus juices	grapefruit, lemons, limes, oranges, satsumas, tangerines, ugli fruit
Mulberry	figs, hops
Palm	coconut, dates, sago
Legumes	beans (all types), black eyed peas, carob, chickpea, gum acacia and tragacanth, kidney beans, lentils, liquorice, peas, peanuts, senna, soya beans, string beans, tamarind
Gourd	courgettes, gherkin, marrow, pumpkin, squashes, water melon
All nuts (different groups)	brazil, cashew, hazel, pistachio, walnut
Potato	pepper (capsicum and chilli), potato, tobacco, tomato
Tropical fruit	banana, pineapple
Sterculia	chocolate, cocoa, cola
Madden	coffee
Tea	tea
Mint	basil, marjoram, mint, oregano, peppermint, sage, savory, spearmint
	all spices and herbs
	all additives and flavourings
	tap water

N.B. The Oligoantigenic diets are for *short*-term use, for example as an exclusion diet. Long-term use is likely to cause deficiencies of vitamins, minerals and other food substances, and encourage allergies to develop to the few foods eaten.

Challenge

The next stage in diagnosing allergy is the challenge. Food allergy is confirmed if a big reduction in symptoms occurs on the exclusion diet. If you suffer from food allergy and you are taking the correct exclusion diet, then an improvement in your health should have started by the eighth day. However, some conditions, like arthritis and eczema, take longer to improve. The arthritis and eczema exclusion diet should be prolonged for 10 or even 14 days.

Having confirmed a food allergy, it is necessary to identify which food is responsible for the allergy. This is done by re-adding excluded foods back into the diet. One new food is added every 2 days. The food challenging is done slowly because there may be a delay of up to 48 hours before a reaction becomes obvious.

There are reactions that occur after a short delay (15 minutes to 4 hours). These include pulse rate change, irritability and headache, lip swelling, vomiting and a runny nose. Urticaria, diarrhoea and asthma are slower to show (delay 1 to 24 hours), and the slowest is usually eczema and arthritis (6 to 48 hours).

When you start a food challenge, you should take a couple of teaspoonful at 12 noon, and then if you get no reaction within an hour, take a good size portion of the food at lunchtime. *Noon* Eat only the food that you are testing. It is *best to* more difficult to tell a food reaction if you start *test* the food at breakfast, since many people feel less than their best in the morning. If you start the new food in the evening, the reaction may occur while you are asleep and be unnoticed. If you have no reaction at lunchtime, then take more of the same food at the evening meal and more the next day. If you suffer no reaction, during these two days then it is a 'safe' food, and can be added to the foods already eaten.

When challenging yourself, it is wise to start

with foods that are least likely to cause an allergic problem (see list page 39). Also you should take foods as single ingredients, for example take wheat as a home-made biscuit rather than bread, which contains yeast and often additives as well as wheat. Fill in the results in the challenge sheet shown below.

If you have a reaction then stop that food immediately and take a tablespoonful of sodium bicarbonate (baking soda) in a pint of spring water. The sodium bicarbonate is a weak alkali and has the power to reduce the allergic reaction. Most allergic reactions make the body more acid, and this acidity is neutralized by the sodium bicarbonate. Your local chemist will be able to supply this substance to you without a prescription. Another helpful remedy is to take 1 gram of vitamin C (wheat-free, milk-free, and yeast-free) with a large glass of water. The vitamin

C helps the body's detoxification processes.

After a reaction you should not challenge yourself with another food for 3 days. If you are unsure as to whether or not you reacted to a food, stop eating it for a week and then re-challenge yourself to the same food. In the interim try other foods. If you re-try the suspect food earlier than a week, the reaction may be 'masked' and consequently not show. Don't forget to challenge yourself with tap water, as it is an increasingly common allergic substance.

You will probably find that different foods will give you different symptoms with a different delay. For example, coffee may give you irritability and headache after a few hours whereas wheat may give you arthritis after 24 hours. Your should remember that most allergies are not fixed and can vary with time. One food that was previously harmless can

Handwritten margin note: Baking Soda

Handwritten margin note: Vit C

Table 2.3 **Results of challenge**

		Reaction (0–4)					
		Day 1			**Day 2**		
Date started	Food taken	a.m.	p.m.	eve	a.m.	p.m.	eve

Table 2.4 **A typical 4 day rotary diet**

Food	Day 1	Day 2	Day 3	Day 4
Protein	Fish	Lamb	Turkey	Rabbit
Fat/Oil	Soya	Sunflower	Olive	Almond
Carbohydrates	Gram flour	Rice	Potato	Buckwheat
Fruit	Melon Pumpkin	Grapes	Banana	Apples/pears
Vegetables	Peas & beans Lentils	Cabbage Cauliflower Sprouts	Celery Carrot Parsnip	Mango Spinach Beetroot
Miscellaneous	Peanuts	Sultanas Raisins	Brazil nuts	Pistachio nuts
Drinks	Pineapple juice	Unfermented grape juice	Banana (liquidized)	Apple or Pear juice

give symptoms, especially after *trigger factors*, such as a virus infection, gastroenteritis, a shock, an operation, or a course of antibiotics.

Be sure to continue filling in your diet diary with your pulse rate and weigh yourself naked both in the morning and last thing at night. When you have an allergic reaction you may find that you fail to drop 1 to 2 pounds overnight because the allergic food causes water retention. Circle any allergy-producing foods in red.

Some people will find that their symptoms disappear on the exclusion diet, but these symptoms do not return even when all the foods have been returned to the diet. This is usually because this individual is not so much allergic to any one food but is made ill by the total load of neotoxins in the food.

Will my food allergy be permanent?

Fortunately, the answer to this question is

usually 'no'. Food allergy reaction can be divided into two types:

a) **Fixed** – this is due to an enzyme defect which is permanent. No matter how long food is avoided it will always cause symptoms when it is taken (e.g. gluten contained in wheat and coeliac disease).

b) **Non-fixed or cyclical** – this is much more common than the fixed kind. Recovery from a non-fixed food allergy can occur, provided the food is avoided and that other allergy producing foods and neotoxins (chemicals, radiation and stress) are kept to a minimum. A food allergy may not reveal itself if the total load of neotoxins is kept low. However, several neotoxins acting together can cause a far greater effect than the sum of their individual effects. The other important factor that encourages a non-fixed allergy to show itself is frequency of exposure to the food. If exposure to food is rare (less than once a week) then a food allergy is unlikely to arise.

Long-term dietary modification

The exclusion diet is a good way to identify your food allergy, but it will cause deficiency diseases if it is the sole form of nutrition long term. In addition, a repetitive restricted diet (like your exclusion diet), is likely to cause food allergies in the long term to the new foods taken.

The answer to this problem is the *rotary diet*, which prevents emergence of new allergies and maintains tolerance to those foods excluded. The easiest way to understand a rotary diet is to see a typical one.

Table 2.4 shows a 4 day rotary diet. After day 4, the diet goes back to day 1 hence the name. The principle is that no food is eaten more frequently than every 4 days, and no 'food family' is repeated more often than every 2 days. (For a full list of 'food families' see page 233.) In order for you to plan your own rotary diets successfully, it is essential to consult this table.

There are a few other important points. Always eat organic foods that have not been processed, sprayed with chemicals, tinned or packaged. Be obsessive about reading labels and finding out the ingredients of everything you eat. Don't forget hidden foods (see page 51). Run your diet day from 4.00pm to 4.00pm, and that way your lunch and evening meal will be in different diet days, and consequently you will have more variety of food in a day.

What are the other methods of detecting food allergy?

There are several other methods of detecting food allergy which are used with varying degrees of success:

- **Skin testing**

  This is useful to detect inhaled substances that cause allergy, e.g. pollens, cat fur, house dust mite and fungi. Unfortunately, this method cannot be used to test for foods.

- **Blood testing**

  In general, blood tests are not helpful in trying to identify food allergies. The 'cytotoxic' test is of limited value and this is carried out by putting white cells from a patient's blood into weak solutions of foods. If the white cells shrivel, that probably indicates a food allergy.

- **Hair testing**

  This is used for mineral content analysis of the body. Sometimes milk allergy is suggested by abnormal calcium and magnesium levels.

- **Applied Kinesiology**

  This is a test that uses principles of acupuncture. The theory of the test is that certain muscle groups become weak when the body is exposed to an allergic food. The weakness is judged by an observer who has to decide if the food has had an adverse effect. This method certainly deserves further study.

- **Provocation/neutralization test**

  This is carried out by injecting food extracts under the skin, or drops of the same into the mouth. Symptoms can be provoked and neutralized (removed) by giving food extracts of the correct dilution.

What are food families?

This is a very useful way of classifying food. All members of a single food family are recognized by the body as being of similar origin. Someone who is allergic to one food is likely to be allergic to other members of the same food family. For example, wheat is a grass, and other members of the same food family include corn, barley, oats and rye. If you are allergic to wheat you are also likely to be allergic to corn, barley, oats and rye, the grasses grown in the western hemisphere.

As a general rule, however, the further away the food is grown from your home, the less likely you are to be allergic to it. Consequently, though bamboo shoots, millet, sorghum and rice are also grasses, they are grown in the eastern hemisphere and you are unlikely to be allergic to them. A full list of food families is given on page 233. This list is invaluable in designing exclusion and rotary diets.

What are hidden foods?

If you are on a milk-free, wheat-free, gluten-free or egg-free diet, you will often have problems because these substances are 'hidden', i.e., undeclared or disguised ingredients of a very wide variety of common foods. The following lists will assist you to decide which foods are safe and which are not.

Hidden Foods: cows' milk

The following list gives the common sources of cows' milk. Occasionally, you may find that one of the following has no milk in it but if in doubt, it is better to leave it out.

Hidden Foods: Cows' Milk

Baby cereals	Chocolates
Baking powder	Chocolate drinks
Biscuits	Chocolate mixtures
Baker's bread	Coffee creamer
Blancmange	Condensed milk
Bologna	Cream
Breakfast cereals	Creamed foods
Butter	Cream sauces
Buttermilk	Creamed soups
Butter sauces	Crisps (some
Caesin	varieties)
Caesinate	Curds
Cakes	Custards
Calcium caesinate	Doughnuts
Cheeses (all forms)	Eggs (scrambled)

Evaporated milk	Pie crust
Foods prepared au gratin	Popcorn
Foods fried in batter, butter, flour mixtures, fritters	Prepared food mixes for biscuits, cakes and puddings
Gravy	Puddings
Hamburgers	Rarebits
Ice cream	Rusks
Homoeopathic tablets	Salad dressings
Junket	Sausages
Mashed potatoes	Sherbets
Malted milk	Skimmed milk
Ovaltine	Sodium caesinate
Lactose	Souffles
Meat loaf	Soups
Margarines	Sweets and confectionery
Milk chocolate	Vegetables canned in sauces
Milk in all forms	Whey
Omelette	Whey protein
Pancakes	White sauce
Pasta	Yoghurt

N.B.: Milk is present in a surprising variety of foods.

Hidden foods: Wheat

The following is a list of common sources of wheat. Occasionally, you will find that one of the following has no wheat in it, but if in doubt, it is better to leave it out. This list is of particular interest to coeliac patients, who are allergic to the gluten found in wheat. Coeliac sufferers must completely avoid ordinary wheat, though they may take gluten-free wheat products without harm. However, most wheat allergic patients will get a reaction when eating gluten-free foods.

Hidden Foods: Wheat

Baked beans	Bread (all types)
Baking powder	Breakfast cereals
Biscuits	Cakes
Bran	Cheese spreads

Chocolate (drinking)
Chocolates
Chutney
Coffee (instant)
Curry powder
Custards
Fish (tinned)
Fish (battered and breadcrumbs)
Fish paste
Flour
Fruit pie filling
Garlic salt
Gravy browning
Horlicks
Ice cream
Lemon cheese
Lemon curd
Margarines
Mayonnaise
Meat pies
Meat (tinned and processed)

Milk shake flavourings
Mincemeat
Mousse
Mustard
Noodles
Ovaltine
Packet seasoning
Pasta
Pastry
Peanut butter
Pepper compounds
Potato (instant)
Puddings
Rye bread
Sauces
Sausages
Savoury spreads
Semolina
Soups
Soya sauce
Stock cubes
Stuffings

Suet (packed)
Sweets
Vegetables (tinned in sauces)

Vegetable salad
Wheat germ

Hidden Foods: Egg

The following list gives the common sources of egg. Occasionally, you may find one of the following has no egg in it, but if in doubt leave it out:

Butter
Biscuits
Cakes
Egg noodles
Lemon curd
Malted milk drinks
Mayonnaise

Pasta
Pastry
Prepared food mixes, biscuits and puddings
Puddings
Soups

What can I use instead of cows' milk and wheat?

Below is a list of foods that can be substituted for cows' milk and wheat. These will enable you to have a more varied diet.

Table 2.5 Substitutes for cows' milk and wheat

Food	Substitutes	Comments
Cows' milk (and cheeses)	Goats' } milk and Sheeps' } cheese	Sometimes causes allergy problems
Cows' milk (and cheeses)	Soya milk	Soya allergy quite common
Wheat	Arrowroot	Useful for gravy and sauce
Wheat	Buckwheat	Useful for spaghetti
Wheat	Sweet chestnut flour	Useful for biscuits and cakes
Wheat	Gram flour from pulses (lentils)	Useful for breads and batters
Wheat	Maize	Useful for biscuits, bread and cakes
Wheat	Potato (fecule and farina)	Useful for baking and thickening

What are organic foods?

Organic fruit and vegetables are those grown without pesticides or fertilizers, other than untreated manure. In addition, no chemicals are used during storage, transport, retail or cooking. Organic sheep and cattle are grazed on organic grass which has been grown without pesticides or fertilizers. The sheep and cattle are given no antibiotics, hormones, or pesticide treated grains. Organic poultry is fed on organically produced grain, free of antibiotics, colourings, hormones and pesticides.

Do different races have the same susceptibility to food allergy?

There are large racial differences in ability to process certain foods. For example, caucasians are able to take large amounts of milk and milk products as adults without difficulty. In contrast, people from Africa, Arabia and Asia are unable to drink large amounts of milk products as adults. These races are able to drink milk as children, however, the enzyme lactase (present in the bowel to digest milk) disappears in adult life. Consequently, if non-European races drink more than a few ounces of milk as an adult they get abdominal pain and distension, and diarrhoea.

Another racial variation is that Japanese and Chinese have a very low tolerance to alcohol. It appears that their liver has less ability to process this substance. Consequently, they become intoxicated on a small amount of alcohol that would have much less effect on a Caucasian.

What effect do bowel flora have on allergies?

The bowel is normally filled with billions of yeasts and bacteria that, in health, exist in a self-regulated balance. Their function is to produce vitamins and act as an initial first stage in the detoxification process. Their chemical flexibility is remarkable, and they are able to break down almost any molecule thrown at them.

As a result, there are major consequences when the bowel flora are altered. The common factors causing an alteration in bowel flora include drugs and diet:

- *Antibiotics* – especially broad-spectrum antibiotics given for a protracted period;
- *Steroids* – hydrocortisone, prednisone and also the steroids in the oral contraceptive;
- *Sugar* – excess sugar and carbohydrates encourage growth of yeast;
- *Alcohol and yeast containing foods* – encourage growth of yeasts.

Any factor that changes the gut flora is likely to produce the following:

- *Intralumenal change*: loss of the normal detoxification capability and vitamin production causes production of gas, diarrhoea and poisons such as acetaldehyde;
- *Bowel wall changes*: the build up of poisons in the lumen of the bowel damages the cells of the gut, which no longer dissolve certain important nutrients and fail to keep out undigested foods and other poisons normally excluded.
- *Body changes*: the immune system and liver detoxification system become overwhelmed with undigested food molecules which are recognized as 'foreign' and attacked. Poisons like acetaldehyde are dissolved in levels greater than can be detoxified; other 'rogue' molecules have hormone-like effects and many even effect DNA and other proteins.

WATER

Water can induce environmental illness in a variety of ways:

- **Infections**

  Water-borne infections are becoming more, rather than less, common. These occur in drinking water, rivers and on beaches. They will be dealt with in greater depth later in this chapter (p. 57).

- **'Normal' water processing**

  During domestic water processing chemicals are added, including aluminium salts, chlorine and fluoride. The section in this chapter will look at the effects of chemicals that are deliberately added to water (see below).

- **Water contaminants**

  These are chemicals that have found their way into the water by accident. The sources of these chemicals include industrial manufacturing processes, agricultural chemicals and the lining of water pipes. These will be dealt with comprehensively in the chemical neotoxin chapter (see Chapter 3).

How is domestic water processed?

Rainwater is collected in reservoirs for storage. It is filtered mechanically and run into settling tanks. Aluminium salts are then added as a 'fining agent' to get rid of the remaining biological matter (algae and plants) which drop out of suspension. The water then passes along to the chemical plant, where chlorine is added to kill bacteria, and in most cases fluoride is added for prevention of tooth decay.

The concentration of chlorine in tap water is very variable, becoming less with time, standing in the pipe and with the distance that the water has to travel from the treatment plant. However, enough chlorine is put in at the treatment plant so that the furthest house, possibly 10 miles away from the water treatment plant, will have adequately chlorinated water even after an overnight wait

in the pipes. This means that a house 100 yards away from a station, is receiving grossly over-chlorinated water.

Aluminium salts added to water have been found to encourage the development of pre-senile dementia (Alzheimer's disease).

Occasionally a pesticide is deliberately added to the water in order to remove a fresh water shrimp that lives in the pipes. Although some people with fish ponds are warned of the impending addition of pesticide to the water, regrettably, no warning is given to pregnant mothers and children, who are most vulnerable to such substances.

As well as 'water-purification' chemicals that are deliberately added, most tap water also contains unacceptably high levels of contaminants, including pesticides, nitrates and organic solvents like trichlorethylene. Despite the water companies' protests that their water is completely 'safe', there are an increasing number of allergic people who have to stay on pure spring water from glass bottles in order to remain well.

INFECTION

Infections are important in Environmental Medicine because, although they are not allergies themselves, they can frequently trigger allergies. Bowel infections in infants are the commonest cause of allergies starting in children aged 0 to 2 years. Infections trigger allergies by damaging enzyme systems and making cell membranes more permeable, overloading the immune and detoxification systems, which in an allergic patient are already busy trying to deal with neotoxins (see Figure 2).

Allergic symptoms commence when the total load of neotoxins exceeds the threshold of the immune and detoxification systems ability to cope. The total load, however, varies unpre-

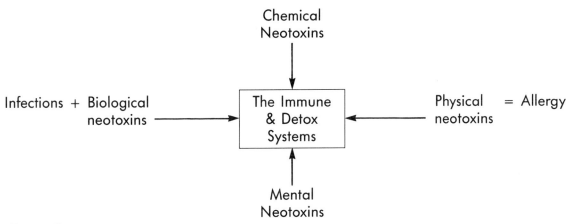

Figure 2

dictably from day to day, thus explaining the variability of allergic symptoms (see Table 2.6).

There are two ways of avoiding infections. In general you should reduce your *total load of neotoxins*. This reduces the burden on your immune and detoxification systems and improves your general health, making you much more able to fight infections successfully.

Specifically, alter your lifestyle so that you reduce your exposure to infections as much as possible. The following section will give you details about some of the more important infections, concentrating on infections from food, water and occupational exposure.

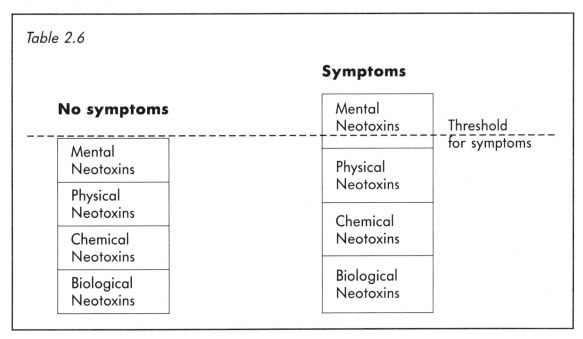

Table 2.6

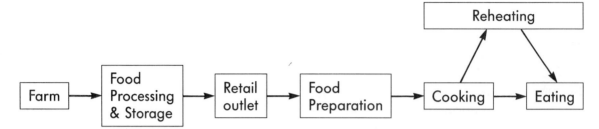

Why do food infections occur?

Foodborne infections occur because of some loss of quality in the food-handling process. Regrettably, these are becoming more, rather than less common, in spite of advanced technology, and the incidence of food poisoning is rising rapidly.

Food infections can arise at any stage of the food production process between farm and dining table. Infection is more common in animal products. Many infections arise as a direct result of intensive farming methods which allow disease to become endemic. Common food-borne infections also appear at the preparation and cooking stages. Inadequate hygiene and use of defective microwave ovens allow infections and toxins to remain in food, with a consequent rise in food poisoning.

Another factor increasing the likelihood of foodborne infections is the use of medicines that reduce stomach acidity (e.g. antacid mixtures and anti-ulcer drugs). Under normal conditions the stomach is very acid (pH 0–1), due to the secretion of hydrochloric acid, which kills almost all bacteria. Antacid mixtures and anti stomach-ulcer drugs reduce the acidity (to pH 4) and this allows some bacteria that would normally have been killed to survive and cause food poisoning.

What are the important infections spread by food?

Salmonella

This is a serious infection present in an alarmingly high proportion of chickens and eggs. Salmonella is killed by adequate cooking. However, the spread of salmonella illustrates some of the main errors that commonly occur in food preparation and cooking. Food is inadequately thawed before cooking (common with deep frozen chickens), and inadequately cooked (common with microwave ovens). Cooked food can also be contaminated with germs from raw food if the two are not handled separately. A further problem may arise if food is allowed to stand after cooking (during which time bacterial multiplication ocurs), and is reheated after standing. You can catch salmonella from raw or undercooked eggs. Raw eggs are often used to make mayonnaise.

Campylobacter

This infection is a much commoner infection than salmonella, and occurs in contaminated meat and water. Regrettably, at the time of writing, most chickens are infected with campylobacter. Fortunately, the infection sustained is relatively mild but will still be a burden on the immune system. The campylobacter germ can be killed by adequate thawing and cooking.

Listeria

This infection is of particular importance to pregnant women, since it can cause miscarriages and stillbirths. It is found in soft cheeses, (brie, camembert), cooked meat, (especially poultry), ice cream and cook-chill foods.

Cook-chill is a food preparation method

very commonly used in hospitals, where the food is frozen immediately after cooking. At a later stage it is reheated, often in a microwave oven. The listeria germ is unusual in that it can grow at low temperatures (2°–6°) similar to those found in refrigerators and storage cabinets for cook-chill foods.

Botulism

This is caused by a toxin produced by the clostridium botulinum germ. The germ is found in soil and usually affects canned goods that have been defectively processed.

Bovine Spongioform Encephalitis (BSE)

This is a recently discovered 'slow' virus infection affecting cows' brains, which become blown up like sponges, (hence the name). There is a very long incubation period (several years), between a cow being infected and becoming ill (hence the term 'slow' virus). Cows' brains in the past were used to make meat pies and hamburgers. There is concern that BSE may be transmitted to humans, but because of the very long incubation period we do not know for certain at present.

Fungal infection of food

In damp conditions, some foods, especially cereals, become infected with fungi. A small percentage of fungi, e.g. aspergillus and fusarium, produce substances called aflatoxins, which are very poisonous. The way to avoid aflatoxins is not to eat mouldy food, especially if the moulds are reddish or brownish. Also you should avoid storing food in damp places, e.g. basements or defrosting fridges.

What are the important waterborne infections?

Leptospirosis

This is a serious infection and may be caught from dirty water, e.g. sewage systems, canals and stagnant pools. The germ can enter the body through cuts, grazes or even via the eyes and mouth.

Cryptosporidiosis

This is a parasite that lives in surface water, swimming pools, and in farm animals, which causes a food-poisoning-like illness. It is not killed by chlorination.

Algal blooms on reservoirs

Algae may combine with bacteria to produce a very poisonous toxin called microcystin. This can cause liver damage in humans and death in smaller animals.

Coliform and other faecal infections

Inadequate arrangements for disposal of sewage have caused many rivers and beaches to have unacceptably high levels of bacteria that constitute a health hazard.

Legionella

Legionnaire's Disease is caused by the legionella germ, which likes to live in warm water (20° to 40°C). This germ is sometimes found in the air conditioning and humidifying systems of large buildings. Such systems, if infected, will then spray an 'aerosol' of legionella bacteria over the occupants.

As with most infections, it is the very young, the old and those whose immune system is not working properly who will first become ill. A healthy person often shows no symptoms to minor infections, although the immune system will be put under strain.

Which occupational groups are exposed to particular hazards of infection?

People who come into contact with animals, hospital specimens, dirty water, soil and sewage are at a greater risk of sustaining

Table 2.7 **Showing serious infections that may be sustained by occupational groups**

Occupation or Recreation	Disease
Workers handling unsterilized bone, hide or hair	Anthrax
Farmers, slaughterhouse workers and vets	Brucellosis
Hospital workers especially laboratory workers, nurses doctors and paramedics	Hepatitis B
Sewage and canal workers, plumbers, farmers, slaughterhouse workers, vets, water sportsmen, anglers	Leptospirosis
Farmers, wool processors and vets	'Q' Fever
Workers in contact with birds	Psittacosis
Farmers and cat lovers	Toxoplasma

infections. Table 2.7 lists occupational and recreational groups more likely to sustain an infection by virtue of their work or hobbies.

Specific measures to avoid these infections:

- Wear protective clothing and follow accepted safety procedures, e.g. hospital workers wear gloves when dealing with human excretions and blood products;
- If you cut yourself, wash well and cover immediately with a waterproof dressing;
- Don't expose yourself to any unnecessary hazard, e.g. swimming in water known to be infected or polluted;
- Avoid these occupations during pregnancy. It will be two people that get infected rather than one;
- Seek medical advice as soon as abnormal symptoms occur, e.g. temperature, swelling, pain, jaundice.

ANIMAL AND PLANT PROTEINS

Animal and plant proteins may cause allergic reactions because allergic processes cause the release of the irritant histamine. Histamine release occurs when the plant or animal protein neotoxin (e.g. pollen, cats fur, house dust mite or fungal spores) reacts with the IgE antibody which is attached to the outside of a mast cell. The pollen-IgE combination causes the mast cell to release histamine which causes:

- Swelling (of the eyes in hayfever);
- Leakage of fluid from blood vessels (runny nose in hayfever);
- Irritation (sneezing in hayfever, wheezing in asthma).

Pollen + | Mast | = Histamine = Allergic
+ IgE | Cell | reaction

Animal and plant protein neotoxins are

particularly important because they cause hayfever, allergic rhinitis and sometimes asthma. These diseases will be dealt with in greater depth in Chapter 7.

SUMMARY

- In the late-twentieth century, food and water pollution is becoming increasingly common and this is causing a rapid rise in the rate of food allergy.
- You are what you eat. If you eat junk food then you are much more likely to suffer from allergies.
- Many food allergies arise because of the repetitive nature of the diet, with high daily levels of common foods like milk, wheat, eggs, tea, coffee, cocoa and citrus fruits.
- Food additives can often be responsible for a wide variety of allergic symptoms, and ideally should be completely excluded from the diet.
- Most packaged foods have their ingredients listed on the side of the packet or tin. However, milk, wheat, eggs and food additives often occur as 'hidden' ingredients of a very wide variety of common foods.
- To find the food responsible for an allergy, try eating an exclusion diet for 1 week, keeping a diet diary during this time. If you improve, challenge yourself with one new food every 2 days in order to identify the allergic culprit.
- Food allergy may be permanent but is usually reversible, and tolerance returns if a food is completely removed from the diet for 6 months or longer. Once this state of tolerance is established, the food can be eaten occasionally (once a week) without symptoms. If, however, it is taken too often (every day) then food allergy will return.
- If you are allergic to one member of a food family (e.g. potato), then you are much more likely to be allergic to other members of the same food family (e.g. tomatoes).
- Whenever possible, eat organic food, that has been grown without pesticides, fertilizers, hormones and antibiotics, since this is much less likely to cause allergy.
- It is important to have normal bowel flora to be healthy. Long term intake of antibiotics, steroids and excess sugar or yeast can have major health consequences.
- Infections frequently trigger allergies. Bowel infections in babies are the ones most likely to cause allergy and should be avoided whenever possible.
- Repetitive exposure to plant and animal proteins can trigger allergic reactions and these proteins should be avoided whenever possible.

CHAPTER THREE

CHEMICALS AND YOUR HEALTH

Imagine a new version of *The Sorcerer's Apprentice* in which the apprentice, instead of being given a mop and bucket, is given a chemistry set. The apprentice tries a bit of magic from the sorcerer's book of spells, but, unfortunately, the chemicals start to multiply and get totally out of hand, filling the atmosphere with poisonous fumes. This is a good analogy for the chemical mess the industrialized world is in. We are waiting for the sorcerer to return and clean up the disaster with a wave of his magic wand, but, unfortunately, this will not happen; it is up to us to start putting our own house in order and change the way we live.

Chemical pollution is an area in which we must *think globally but act locally*. Chemical fumes don't just stay where they are created or sprayed. Alarming tests have shown that when pesticide is sprayed in North Africa on a Monday, some of it reaches Florida by Wednesday and another portion reaches London after a further delay. There are now 350,000,000 cars in the world and factories all round the globe are releasing fumes and making products, such as paints, glues, plastics, aerosols and solvents, which release chemicals into the atmosphere. We are reaching (or have passed) the planet's capacity to recycle all these chemicals. The good news, however, is that what is good for the individual is also good for the planet. By reducing your own *total load of neotoxins* you are doing the best possible thing to reverse the downward spiral. Failure to stop the chemical pollution of air, food and water will cause a drop in life expectancy. This has already occurred in highly polluted areas in Russia and Eastern Europe where the average citizen lives to only 40 years.

The problems caused by the chemicals are more accurately called sensitivities rather than allergies, though the latter term is still frequently used. Chemical sensitivities usually start because of one particular source of chemicals, for example car fumes. If this neotoxin is not removed then the body starts to react to other chemicals as well. These are called 'cross-sensitivities'. If exposure continues, the number of cross-sensitivities increases still further until the body reacts to almost every food and chemical in the environment. At this stage the person is called a 'universal reactor'.

Chemical sensitivity can be triggered by two sorts of chemical events:

● **Acute massive exposure**
 This may occur after an industrial accident (*reported* events include Bhopal in India, Soweso in Italy and Flixborough in England), chemical application and handling (e.g. pesticide-spraying or

chemical spill), or wartime exposure (mustard gas, nerve gas, agent orange). If you experience an acute massive exposure to chemicals sensitivity may persist permanently after the exposure.

● **Chronic exposure**
Chemical sensitivities usually start because of chronic exposure to a chemical neotoxin, e.g. formaldehyde. The standard, but *incorrect* advice, is that there can be no danger because the concentration of the chemical is below the officially recognized danger level; but this has been set at a far too high level.

Safe levels

The 'safe' level of a chemical is often completely wrong because of four fundamental errors in the testing processes.

1. **Wrong individuals tested**
Chemical toxicity testing is carried out on healthy volunteers (usually young men), when those most susceptible are the very young or old, pregnant women and those already ill. Other toxicity tests carried out on laboratory animals, e.g. rats, yield questionable results because of major differences between human and other mammals' metabolism; rats, for example, can make their own vitamin C.

2. **Acute testing but chronic exposure**
The toxicity testing is usually carried out over a relatively short period despite many individuals' chronic exposure. A chronic exposure allows chemicals to bio-accumulate, so that after many years they may reach dangerous levels and cause symptoms.

3. **Individual variation ignored**
There is enormous individual variation from person to person in the ability to detoxify any chosen chemical. A standard

dose of chemical that has no obvious effect on one person will make another very ill (e.g. think, for example, of the different effect of alcoholic drinks on different people). Individuals who have defective detoxification systems are much more likely to suffer from chemical sensitivity.

4. **'The cocktail effect'**
In the real world we are exposed to hundreds of different chemicals every day. A chemical on its own may be relatively harmless, but when mixed with other commonly occurring chemicals may cause an interaction that makes it much more toxic, for example the combination of alcohol and tranquillizers.
    Another problem is that many organic chemicals are bound to body fat, and over time the amount stored goes up (bio-accumulation). The body is often not able to excrete the chemical in the times between exposures, and thus the level continually goes up over your whole lifetime. Chronic exposure is particularly likely to be a problem if your *total load of neotoxins* is also high.

WHAT HAPPENS WHEN I AM EXPOSED TO A CHEMICAL NEOTOXIN?

On the initial exposure to a chemical neotoxin, you will usually suffer an 'alarm reaction' (see page 33). The chemical can be smelt, and common symptoms include light-headedness, headache and palpitations.

If the exposure continues, the adaption phase (see page 33) is entered, and a sense of smell for that chemical is lost. Surprisingly, instead of feeling unwell, continuing exposure to the chemical, will probably give you a 'lift' (e.g. glue sniffing). If exposure then ceases, as the level of the chemical in the body drops, then withdrawal symptoms begin.

If, instead of removing the chemical, exposure continues, eventually you will reach the 'exhaustion stage' (see page 33), and instead of a chemical giving you a 'lift', you will feel immediately worse at each new exposure. By this time there may well be permanent damage to the body.

HOW DOES THE BODY USUALLY DETOXIFY NEOTOXINS?

The normal detoxification process takes place all over the body, but especially in the liver, and consists of two phases illustrated in Figure 3.1. Phase I is called the cytochrome 450 redox enzyme system and occurs in the endoplasmic reticulum part of the cell. It converts a neotoxin (arbitrarily called X) firstly to an alcohol (with the OH group), then to an aldehyde (with CHO group), and finally to an acid (with the H group) which can then be excreted via the kidney into the urine.

The neotoxin either enters the phase II pathway directly or else entry from phase I as an aldehyde (with a CHO group). In phase II, which occurs throughout the cell substance, a sugar, amino acid, or other molecule is added or conjugated to the neotoxin to make it less toxic so that it can be excreted via the liver into the bile, or via the kidney into the urine.

Phase I and phase II of the detoxification process can work properly only if there are adequate vitamins, minerals, amino acids and fatty acids available in the cell. In addition, the detoxification enzyme symtems must not be overloaded or poisoned by any factor in the air, food or water. If the normal detoxification pathways fail to operate, then abnormal detoxification pathways are opened up.

The most common abnormal detoxification pathways are illustrated in Figure 3.2. These pathways are followed when the usual pathways are blocked (marked 'Pathways blocked'); then metabolites become backlogged and this increased concentration of toxic substances causes allergies.

When the conversion of the neotoxin (X) into a neotoxin alcohol (XOH) is blocked, then a neotoxin epoxide (X=O) is produced. This is a highly reactive and dangerous metabolite that causes many allergy symptoms, especially affecting the brain, and even increasing the risk of cancer.

When the conversion of the neotoxin alcohol (X=OH) to neotoxin aldehyde is blocked, then chloral hydrate ($CCl_3.CH(OH)_2$) is produced, which has a toxic effect on the brain. When the metabolism of neotoxin aldehyde is blocked then aldehyde (CHO) builds up, which causes a large number of symptoms, including damage to cells and the detoxification system, the destruction of important substances like vitamins, and the creation of 'orphan' chemicals that can't be broken down.

HOW CAN MY DOCTOR TELL IF MY DETOXIFICATION SYSTEM IS WORKING?

Allergies will strongly suggest that the detoxification system is not working properly, but most conventional blood tests give little or no indication that the detoxification system has a problem until it is on the verge of collapse. There are some blood tests that can give you an indication of whether detoxification system damage has occurred. The substances measured include:

- **Free Radical Quenching Enzyme**
  Enzymes such as superoxide dismutase (SOD) and glutathione peroxidase have the job of stopping backlogged or 'orphan' metabolites and free radicals from punch-

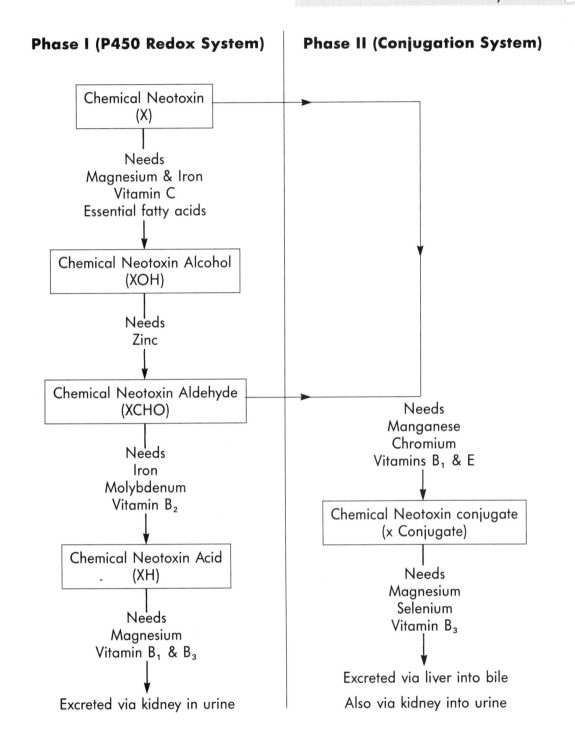

Phase I (P450 Redox System)

Phase II (Conjugation System)

Chemical Neotoxin
(X)

Needs
Magnesium & Iron
Vitamin C
Essential fatty acids

Chemical Neotoxin Alcohol
(XOH)

Needs
Zinc

Chemical Neotoxin Aldehyde
(XCHO)

Needs
Iron
Molybdenum
Vitamin B_2

Chemical Neotoxin Acid
(XH)

Needs
Magnesium
Vitamin B_1 & B_3

Excreted via kidney in urine

Needs
Manganese
Chromium
Vitamins B_1 & E

Chemical Neotoxin conjugate
(x Conjugate)

Needs
Magnesium
Selenium
Vitamin B_3

Excreted via liver into bile

Also via kidney into urine

Figure 3.1 **Normal Detoxification Pathways**

ing holes in cell membranes, setting off a cascade of damage. Reduced levels of these two enzymes indicate that the detoxification system is failing.

- **Markers of Tissue Damage**
  If free radicals manage to damage the cell membranes they release lipid peroxides. A raised level of lipid peroxides indicates cell damage due to the inability of the

detoxification system to cope with the build up of metabolites and free radicals.

- **Raised Metabolite Levels**
  If the detoxification system has to process increased amounts of neotoxins, then it will produce increased D-glucaric acid, mercapturic acid and formic acid, one or all of which will be raised.

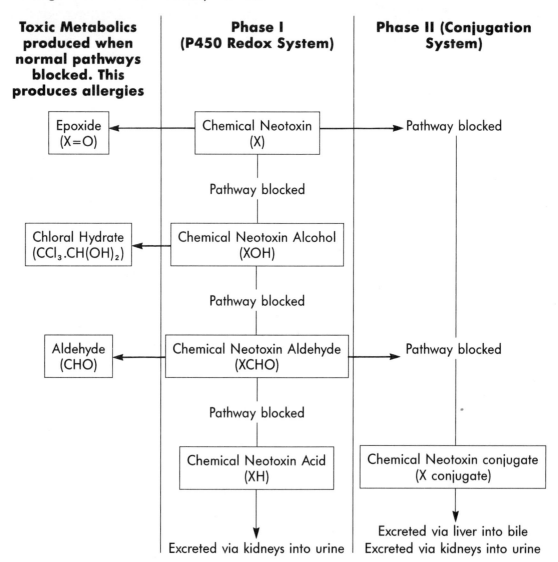

Figure 3.2 **Abnormal Detoxification Pathways**

Localized symptoms

Brain: (commonest organ affected by chemicals) headache, reduced concentration and memory, 'high', irritability, feeling 'doped up' or drowsy, 'hangover-like' feeling, addictions (e.g. glue sniffing)

Nose: heightened or reduced sense of smell

Heart: palpitations

Lung: asthma

Generalized symptoms

tired all the time
fatigue
muscular weakness

swelling of many parts of the body including eyelids, lips and mouth, hands and fingers, abdomen and ankles

sweating (intermittent)

overweight,
underweight
or having a rapidly changing weight

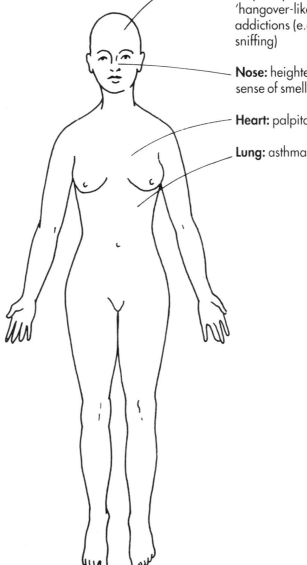

Figure 3.3 **Common symptoms of chemical sensitivity**

HOW CAN I TELL IF I HAVE A CHEMICAL SENSITIVITY?

You are likely to get symptoms as described in Chapter 1 (page 20), however, there are particular features that will suggest you have a chemical sensitivity.

- You may have many symptoms, especially headache, fatigue, reduced concentration and memory, muscle weakness, irritability, excitability and feeling 'doped up'. Any or all of these symptoms are likely to come on after the initial exposure, or else during the hangover.
- You are likely to be chemically sensitive to several different groups of substances, e.g. combustion fumes, solvent fumes, plastic fumes, formaldehyde, alcohol and antibiotics.
- You will probably feel worse in one particular place, e.g. in the kitchen, or at one particular time, e.g. on Mondays when returning to work, on long car journeys. Often other people will feel unwell in the same place.
- You feel better outdoors and in well ventilated places.
- You either intensely dislike, or paradoxically are very fond of, chemical fumes, e.g. petrol fumes, tar fumes, glue and paint fumes.
- You are likely either to have a very acute sense of smell or to have lost your sense of smell completely.

WHAT FACTORS MAKE ME MORE LIKELY TO SUFFER FROM A CHEMICAL SENSITIVITY?

A high total load of neotoxins

If your load of neotoxins from *all* sources, i.e. biological neotoxins (food, water, and infection), chemical neotoxins, physical neotoxins (electromagnetic radiation, and sound) and mental neotoxins (stress, exposure to shocks and accidents) is high then you're more likely to suffer a chemical sensitivity. It is the *total* load that is important, since that governs how much reserve your immune and detoxification systems have left.

Your individual susceptibility

This is dependent on your age, your sex, your racial background and the genes that you inherited from your parents. As a general rule, young children and old people have less resistance to most problems. Adult women seem to be about twice as likely as men to suffer from allergies (see Chapter 15), although before puberty allergies seem to be commoner amongst boys.

There is a large genetic variation in the ability to withstand exposure to chemicals. This is related to the activity of liver and other enzymes systems. Some people produce defective enzymes and, consequently, the body is not able to process certain neotoxins, making such individuals much more susceptible to chemical sensitivities. There is no obvious outward sign that susceptible people have a problem. However, the speed at which an individual can break down a standard dose of the drug debrisoquine gives a good idea of the individual's resistance to chemical sensitivity.

Your resources for recovery

Recovery to most insults can be achieved with sleep and rest, exercise, (with saunas), to encourage loss of toxins through sweat, and appropriate vitamins and mineral supplements (see Chapter 6).

HOW DO CHEMICALS ENTER THE BODY?

Chemicals enter the body through three routes, being eaten, being inhaled or by contact with the skin.

Chemical neotoxins in food and drink

There are many contaminants in food and water. They have got in by accident or by bad practice. These chemicals are absorbed through the bowel, which has a surface area of 400 square metres, and may then affect any organ.

Common chemical contaminants in food include halocarbon and hydrocarbon solvents, insecticides, herbicides and fungicides, antibiotics, hormones and steroids, petrochemical fuels, oils and waxes and their breakdown products, metals and plastics from cooking utensils. Phenolic compounds including tin can linings, formaldehyde compounds, natural gas and other gases.

Chemical contaminants in tap water include halocarbons and hydrocarbon solvents, other halocarbons, including PCB, insecticides, herbicides and fungicides, nitrates and other fertilizers, heavy metals including lead, mercury, cadmium, aluminium, copper, arsenic, polyvinyl chloride, sex steroids, asbestos, infections from sewage, disposal and contamination by animal manures and household waste, and toxic gases such as sulphur dioxide.

There is an effect called *bioconcentration* that occurs with chemicals that are stored in body fat, e.g. pesticides. The result of this effect is that these substances become more

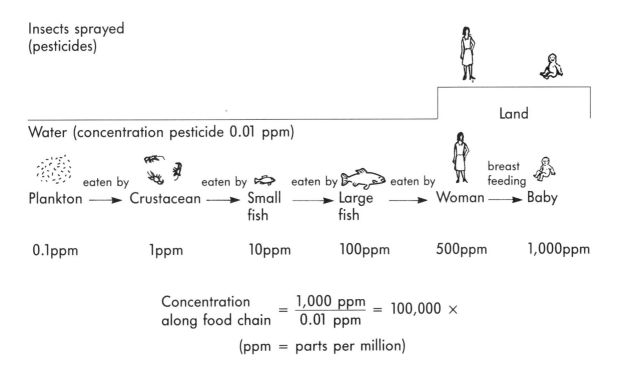

Insects sprayed
(pesticides)

Land

Water (concentration pesticide 0.01 ppm)

Plankton → Crustacean → Small fish → Large fish → Woman → Baby

eaten by / eaten by / eaten by / eaten by / breast feeding

0.1ppm   1ppm   10ppm   100ppm   500ppm   1,000ppm

$$\frac{\text{Concentration}}{\text{along food chain}} = \frac{1{,}000 \text{ ppm}}{0.01 \text{ ppm}} = 100{,}000 \times$$

(ppm = parts per million)

Figure 3.4 **Bioconcentration along a food chain (× 100,000)**

Pesticides

concentrated as they pass up the food chain. Since humans are always at the top of food chains (no animal eats humans), we are the people who most experience the result of this phenomenon. The concentrating effect along a food chain can be as much as 100,000 times! Breast milk, which is largely an emulsion of fat, further concentrates poisons stored in fats, which is why it is so important for a nursing mother to have an unpolluted diet. A typical example of the bioconcentration is shown in Figure 3.4.

The way to avoid chemical contamination of food is to eat organic food, failing that, natural food, but certainly avoid junk food. The way to avoid chemical contamination of water is to drink a recommended spring water from a safe source in glass bottles. There are other ways of purifying water. However, the method chosen depends on which contaminants that you are trying to remove. Table 3.1 lists the commonly used sources and methods with their strength and weaknesses. No single process is best for all problems.

Table 3.1 **Sources and methods of purification of water**

Sources of water or purification method	Principle used for purification	Method can avoid or remove	Method fails to remove	Comments
Spring water (bottled in glass)	Filtration through rocks	Chlorine	Nitrates Minerals Pesticides Organisms Particulate matter	Spring water is only as pure as source and bottling method
Shallow well (less than 30' deep)	Filtration through rocks	Chlorine	Nitrates Minerals Pesticides Organisms Particulate matter	Shallow well may be contaminated by ground water and faecal contamination
Deep well (more than 30' deep)	Filtration through rocks	Chlorine	Nitrates Minerals Pesticides Organisms Particulate matter	Less risk of contamination from ground water and faecal contamination. *Caution* – Radon

Sources of water or purification method	Principle used for purification	Method can avoid or remove	Method fails to remove	Comments
				contamination and PCB from submersible pumps
Ceramic & other filters	Filtration	Particulate matter e.g. organisms and asbestos	All dissolved matter, solvents, pesticides	Useful in conjunction with another method. May add pollutants
Activated Charcoal	Filtration	Chlorine, some pesticides some minerals, dissolved gases	Organisms and particles and some organic chemicals	Needs replacing frequently. Can become infected
Reverse Osmosis	Filtration	Pesticides, solvents and organic chemicals and fluorides. All organisms and particulate matter	Chlorine and some dissolved minerals and organic chemicals	Small daily output. Membrane can become blocked and are sometimes made of plastic
Ion Exchange Resin (water softener)	Ion exchange	Chlorine Calcium Carbonate	Organic chemicals. All organisms and Particulate matter	Depends on ion exchange resin used. Some resins are more effective

Sources of water or purification method	Principle used for purification	Method can avoid or remove	Method fails to remove	Comments
Ultra violet light	ultra violet radiation	Organisms	Organic chemicals Chlorine, nitrate minerals and particulate matter	Kills all organisms and without adding chlorine
Boiling for 10 minutes	Heat	Volatile pesticides. All organisms	Non-volatile pesticides and organic chemicals Particulate matter	Useful in an emergency
Distillation (Domestic Models)	Distillation	Some organic chemicals and all minerals, organisms and particulate matter	Some chlorine compounds and other volatile organic chemicals	Often tastes awful! Uses a lot of electricity
Water 'purification' tablets	Chlorination	Organisms	Everything else	Adds more chlorine than usual. Only useful in a desperate emergency

Other water purification tips: Run your water for 2 to 3 minutes if water has stood overnight in pipes. Lead levels can be 100 times normal after overnight standing, especially in soft water areas.

Inhalation

The fastest and commonest way for chemicals to enter the body is through the lungs. The lungs have a very large surface area equivalent to that of half a tennis court (100 square metres). This enables chemicals to enter the blood's circulation within 1 to 2 seconds and to get to the brain in 7 seconds, hence the very rapid effect of airborne chemicals especially on the brain.

Skin contact

The skin provides a large surface area for the absorption of chemicals (1.5 square metres). More than half the chemicals entering the body from water are absorbed through the skin. However, the chemicals that are most easily absorbed through the skin are those that are fat soluble, i.e. most organic chemicals.

WHICH CHEMICALS ARE LIKELY TO CAUSE PROBLEMS WITH MY HEALTH?

There are so many chemicals that it is necessary to have some sort of classification of these substances. A loose classification based on the use of the chemical is far more valuable than a precise but unmanageable scientific classification based on chemical composition. Consequently, there is considerable overlap in the following list.

petrol and diesel and their combustion products
natural gas, other fuels and their combustion products
incinerators
cigarette smoke
solvents and glues, paints and varnishes ('do it yourself')
cleaning fluids and polishes
pesticides (insecticides, herbicides, fungicides)
fertilizers (nitrates)
pharmaceutical drugs
dyes
plastics
synthetic fibres and materials
soaps and detergents
perfumes, cosmetics and deodorants
treated papers, boards and woods (chipboard and plywood)
chlorinated hydrocarbons (halocarbons with C-Cl bond)
toxic gases (sulphur dioxide, oxides of nitrogen, ozone)
toxic metals (lead, mercury, cadmium, arsenic, aluminium)
alcohols (all alcoholic drinks, surgical and methylated spirits)
phenols (dyes, drugs, plastics, preservatives)
terpenes (paint fumes, anaesthetics, hydrocarbon fuel fumes)
formaldehyde (textiles, dyes, foams and rubbers, and *many* others).

Petrol, diesel and their combustion products (motor vehicle fumes)

We are now starting to pay the price for the motor car age. The centres of most large cities are no longer fit for human habitation due to the alarmingly high level of petrol and diesel fumes. Petrol and diesel fumes are amongst the commonest causes of chemical sensitivity, and diesel fuel usually causes more problems than petrol. Pointers that suggest that your chemical sensitivity problem may be due to car fumes include:

● Being ill in cars and buses, especially when sitting in the back with the window open;
● Being unwell when you go into the centre of a town, especially in the rush hour;
● Living near a busy road, especially one with a junction or underpass where car

fumes build up. People living near a busy road have been found to have a raised incidence of cancer.

If you have a chemical sensitivity to vehicle fumes you should move away from a main road to a less busy one. To assess whether or not you are too close to a main road, you should use the general rule that if you can *hear* traffic, then you are too close.

traffic

One of the commonest ways to induce chemical sensitivity is to have a house with an integral garage. The chemical sensitivity arises when exhaust fumes leak into the house. It may also be due to other DIY chemicals kept in the garage. The garage is often used to store paints, solvents, varnishes, glues and cleaners which, even if tightly sealed, still tend to leak a little. Petrol exhaust fumes are hot and, therefore rise; consequently the room above the garage (often a bedroom) becomes filled with these gases. If the occupant of that room also has a poor diet and stressful lifestyle, then a chemical sensitivity is very likely to arise.

garages

The ingredients of traffic fumes are not just hydrocarbons, but also oxides of nitrogen and carbon monoxide. When these gases are exposed to bright sunlight, ozone and free radicals are formed, which once again add to the total load that must be managed by the detoxification system.

Natural gas, paraffin, heating oil and their combustion products (central heating and cooking)

These are used to heat homes, offices and schools. Chemical sensitivity may arise from the unburnt fuels or their combustion products. Some patients are so sensitive to natural gas that there is enough leakage from existing plumbing, even when all devices are turned off, to give them symptoms. The effect of the leakage is made worse because natural gas rises (through being lighter than air) and also it is supplied at higher pressure than the previously used town gas.

An unventilated kitchen is a dangerous place to be. Natural gas combustion fumes contain carbon monoxide and oxides of nitrogen. After a gas cooker has been burning for a couple of hours in an unventilated kitchen, the level of pollution with toxic gases is several times higher than that experienced standing in busy rush hour traffic. This is a very good reason to ensure that all kitchens have adequate ventilation.

Some chemically sensitive people react to food cooked in a gas oven. It is quite common that people with an apparent coffee allergy are not, in fact, allergic to the coffee but to the gas used to roast the coffee beans.

Unburnt paraffin liquid and especially paraffin combustion fumes cause problems in susceptible people. Paraffin fires are usually put in the centre of a room without any proper escape route for the exhaust gases, and toxic fumes which build up to dangerous levels.

Central heating system design and installation often leaves a lot to be desired. The flues are sometimes placed in areas where fumes can leak back into the house. Chemical sensitivity to central heating fumes is usually worse in the winter, and inside the house, and better in the summer and outside the house. The best heating for allergic people is movable electric radiators (providing, of course, that they are not electrically sensitive: see Chapter 4). If a central heating boiler is used it should be sited in a sealed room that does not directly communicate with the house. This prevents leakage of fumes into the house affecting the occupants.

Electric Heat

Incinerators

Incinerators are used to dispose of dangerous chemicals like PCBs and contaminated organic solvents by burning them at high temperatures. Even when they are working properly, residents in surrounding areas are showered with neotoxins and carcinogens. If the incinerator is operated at a lower temperature then horrendously poisonous chemicals like dioxins are produced and this explains the high incidence of allergies and cancer in the proximity of incinerators.

Cigarette Smoking

Smoking is a major cause of ill health and the most important cause of premature death (dying before the age of 65 years) in the western world. Exclusion diets, avoidance of chemicals and other measures in '*the superhealth plan*' (Chapter 6) are of reduced value in smokers or passive smokers (non-smokers breathing in other people's smoke). Cigarettes contain nicotine and tar, both of which have a damaging effect on the immune system. Smoking is an *addiction* and is dealt with in greater depth in Chapter 13.

Solvents and glues, paints and varnishes (do it yourself)

It has long been known that the vapour of solvents and glues, paints and varnishes may bring on an asthma attack. However, any of the above chemicals may be responsible for symptoms of chemical sensitivity. Unless you work with the above chemicals, exposure is usually episodic and easier to relate to a bout of illness. However, highly susceptible individuals will react to very low levels of 'DIY' products e.g. leakage from storerooms and garages. Even the apparently tightly sealed bottles and cans often leak a little.

When you are painting or glueing, you will receive a massive dose of halocarbons (halocarbon = chlorine-carbon bond) solvents. All the solvent must fully evaporate from a glue, paint or varnish for it to harden

into its longlasting form. There is no escape route for the solvent in an enclosed space with poor ventilation, and so the atmospheric concentration builds up rapidly. This solvent is then inhaled and absorbed through the lungs.

Cleaning fluids and polishes

Under this heading is included a wide range of cleaning fluids, carpet and 'dry' cleaners, and a range of wood, floor and metal polishes. These all contain halocarbon solvents which are fat soluble and are absorbed very quickly through the lungs and skin. They have their greatest effect on the brain, which is made largely of fat. Consequently most of the symptoms caused by these substances are mental (e.g. irritability, hyperactivity, depression and muscle weakness).

Pesticides

These substances have been designed to be poisonous in very low concentrations, e.g. 1 to 2 parts per million, and 1 teaspoonful can kill an adult. Plants and animals have great difficulty in breaking down these substances and, consequently, pesticides persist in the environment for many years. Unfortunately, however, the pesticides don't stay where they are sprayed. They travel thousands of miles in air currents, and are leached in to the water supply, at which point they enter the food chain.

They are bioconcentrated along food chains and they bioaccumulate in body fat (see Figure 3.4). There is often a long delay between application to the ground and the side effects of poisoning becoming obvious in the plants and animals in the food chain. Even if the use of pesticides stopped today, it would be another 30 years before we would see the full effect of the pesticides that have already been applied.

There is also the phenomenon of 'synergy'

(a magnification effect) between pesticides. This means that when two pesticides are used together, their combined effect may be 100 times greater than using one or other on its own. Synergy may also occur between a pesticide and its 'inert' base. The deadly dioxin may be present in a pesticide without notification, increasing the poisonous effect on flora, fauna and humans.

The usage of pesticides has increased 5 to 15 times because the pests sprayed have become resistant. However, another problem is that the predators that fed on the pests have also been killed. Despite regulations governing use, there is little *practical* control over how, when and where pesticides are applied. Governments don't routinely measure pesticide levels. This is probably because they would have to take some action when they were found to be too high.

Pesticides can be classified according to their usage.

Pesticides 'bioaccumulate' in body fat. It may be several years of chronic exposure to a pesticide before symtpoms start to appear. The symptoms usually will not start to lessen until detoxification is carried out as described later in this section. The threshold for symptoms can vary daily depending upon general health level.

Insecticides

These are used to kill insects that feed on crops. They are used on *growing* crops, and consequently are likely to be incorporated into the plant tissue. They are also used to treat stored grain. There are four groups of insecticides:

● **organochlorine** – very persistent fat bound pesticide. Many now banned.

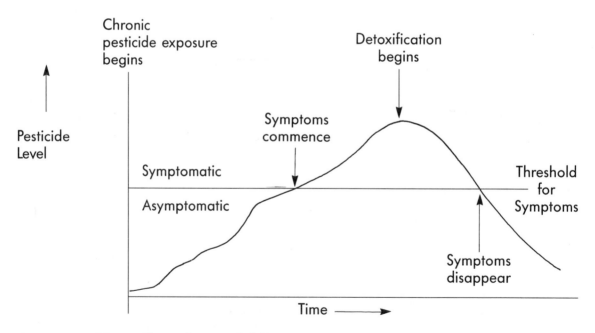

Figure 3.5 **How Chronic Pesticide Exposure causes bioaccumulation and appearance of symptoms**

- **organophosphorous** – derived from nerve gases
- **carbamates** – work in a similar way to organophosphorous compounds
- **pyrethroids** – initially derived from the chrysanthemum plant.

Herbicides

There are two sorts of herbicides:

- non-specific ones, that kill all plant life.
- specific ones that kill broad leaved plants, i.e. weeds, leaving the crop unharmed.

Some herbicides have a similar structure to naturally occurring plant hormones and growth promoters. These are absorbed into the plant and then either block metabolism or wildly overstimulate it, in either case causing plant death.

Fungicides

These kill fungi and they are usually based on a heavy metal, e.g. mercury or copper, or a hydrocarbon compound containing sulphur. They are sprayed on plants, especially fruit, and they are often applied with paraffin to promote penetration into the tissue. At the time of eating traces of fungicides can still be found in food; unfortunately, washing does not remove these chemicals.

Fungicides are also used to preserve wood and kill dry rot. Pentachlorophenol (PCP), is a major health hazard to the workers making and using it. Despite the insistence of building societies and banks on fungicidal treatment of houses, it is often not necessary. Wood used in construction of houses remains strong for up to 500 years providing that it is kept dry and well ventilated. There are now low toxicity fungicides, which have a 10-year life as opposed to the usual 30-year life, and are much less poisonous.

Pesticides work by damaging the cell function of plants or animals. There are five basic mechanisms:

- Disruption of nerve function either at the nerve impulse level or the synapse level.
- Disruption of DNA and RNA function and replication affecting cell division and protein synthesis.
- Disrupting energy release from food, stopping all intracellular metabolic activity.
- Disruption of hormone and growth regulator function causing disturbed patterns and rate of growth.
- Disruption of photosynthesis stopping plant from utilizing energy of sunlight.

Pesticides may pollute air, food or water and consequently may enter the body via:

- Skin or mucous membrane especially eyes. The commonest mode of entry of pesticides is by direct contact with skin.
- Lungs
- Bowels

The following are high risk sources, situations and activities for pesticide exposure:

- All treated wood and timber and all wood workers due to fungicides and wood preservatives.
- Building, decorating and DIY due to pesticide treatment of wood, wallpaper, paint, glue, mortar, masonry and cable.
- New carpets, textiles and clothes, especially wool and cotton due to treatment with insecticides.
- Pets, vets and other animal handlers due to pesticide applications, such as flea collars and dusting powders.
- Agricultural animals and their handlers due to pesticide applications such as sheep dips and cattle dressings.
- Farms, farm workers and both commercial

and domestic gardeners, especially those working in greenhouses and other areas with poor ventilation; also those living and working nearby due to airborne pesticide spread.

- Pest control, both domestic and commercial, of insects, rodents, birds and other vermin, e.g. fly sprays and fumigation.
- Pharmaceutical lotions, shampoos and sprays for treatment and control of scabies, lice, house dust mites, bedbugs and fleas, and organisms responsible for malaria, schistosomiasis and filariasis.
- Spraying of fields, orchards, parks, gardens, roads, pavement, paths, railway tracks, power stations and military establishments with pesticides, especially herbicide. Anyone working or living nearby or walking through or past such sites is at risk.
- Cleaning work in shops, offices, factories and homes.
- Airport runways due to herbicides and aeroplanes due to pesticides used to kill rodents, insects and mosquitoes; also aeroplanes and helicopters used for aerial spraying.
- Water and water treatment for drinking, swimming, recreation and irrigation, crop watering, fish farming in reservoirs, rivers, estuaries, canals and watercourses.
- Treatment of water in factory and office humidifier and air conditioning systems with pesticides to prevent infections like legionella.
- Ships, boats, harbours, jetties, piers and oil rigs treated with anti-fouling paint.
- Sewage and effluent water polluted with pesticides.
- Food processing, transport, storage and retail, due to pesticide residues.
- Manufacturing, transport, storage and retail of pesticides.

Pesticide poisoning is often confused with other illnesses. Acute poisoning may be confused with heat stroke, asthma, gastroenteritis or brain haemorrhage. Chronic poisoning may be confused with a 'persistent cold', a 'flu-like illness' or 'hayfever'. The treatment, which should be carried out by a suitably qualified person is as follows.

Acute pesticide poisoning
N.B: **Wear protective clothing and mask**

- **Resuscitation**
  Airway — Keep clear and remove vomit if necessary.
  Breathing — Give oxygen and artificial respiration.
  Circulation — Check pulse, blood pressure and ECG.
  Other — also check respiration, conscious level and neurological signs.
- **Decontaminate**
  Remove patient from source of pesticide taking off all clothing. Clean skin, hair and nails with soapy water to stop delayed absorption. Wash eyes and mucous membranes well. If pesticide ingested consider inducing vomiting and/or administer intragastric charcoal, followed by gastric lavage and saline cathartic.
- **Antidote**
  Identify pesticide — see label on container. Contact Hospital Poisons Centre.
  Administer appropriate antidote. Anticonvulsant may be necessary.
- **Observation**
  Keep under observation for 24–48 hours and take blood for pesticide level.
- **Notification**
  Report case to your local Health and Safety Executive (see local phone book for number).

Central Nervous and Autonomic
Tired all the time, fatigue, exhaustion, weakness, paralysis, headache, dizziness, nausea, vomiting, tremor, unco-ordination, fits, unsteadiness, numbness, tingling, peripheral neuropathy, blurred vision, contracted pupils, sweating, salivation, fever and temperature regulation problems, CNS depression, coma, brain damage, symptoms that mimic recognized neurological diseases, e.g. multiple sclerosis, Parkinson's and Motor Neurone Disease

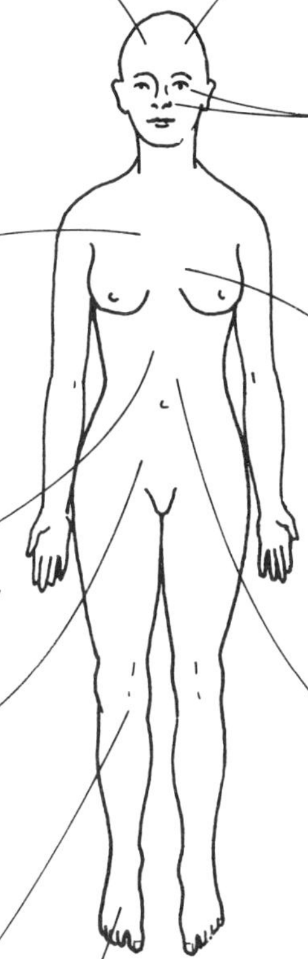

Lungs
Burning and irritation of lungs, difficulty in breathing, shortness of breath, excess secretions from lung, bronchospasm, asthma, respiratory depression, cyanosis, lung damage

Liver detoxification
Disruption of many liver enzyme systems, low tolerance to chemicals and alcohol, chemical hepatitis, jaundice, liver necrosis, liver damage

Urinary and Reproductive
Dysuria and frequency of urination, incontinence, kidney damage, miscarriages and malformations, reduced sperm count, sterility, impotence and loss of libido, pesticides concentrated into breast milk

Musculo-skeletal
Muscular twitching, muscle cramps, muscular tenderness and pains, low strength, fitness and stamina, paralysis, arthritis and rheumatic pains

Skin
Dermatitis especially of hands, skin irritation, itching, blistering and burning, rashes, urticuria, eczema

Psychiatric
Irritability, anxiety, confusion, concentration and memory loss, personality change, emotional problems, insomnia, hallucinations, psychotic illness, lassitude, depression, reduced drive, apathy

Eyes and Ears, Nose and Throat
Burning, irritating and watering mucous membranes of ears, nose and throat, conjunctivitis, rhinitis, sore throat, eye damage

Heart and Cardiovascular
Slow pulse, fast pulse, cardiac arrhythmias, heart block, high blood pressure, low blood pressure, chest pain, circulatory failure, heart muscle damage

Gastro-intestinal
Nausea, vomiting, abdominal pains and cramps, diarrhoea, thirst, dehydration, odd taste in the mouth, loss of appetite, weight loss, blood loss from gastro-intestinal tract

Endocrine
Suppression of adrenal cortex, hypothyroidism, hyperglycaemia, suppression of endocrine function

Cancer
Cancer of all systems especially white cells. Mutagenic, teratogenic and oncogenic effects

Haematological and Immune
Immune system depression, anaemias, white cell depression, clotting problems

Figure 3.6 **Typical symptoms of pesticide poisoning**

Chronic pesticide poisoning

- **Detoxification**

  Advise organic food and bottled spring water diet.

  Advise avoidance of further pesticide exposure. See high risk sources.

  Advise avoidance of all pollutants, e.g. car fumes.

  Give adequate vitamins and mineral supplements.

  Recommend saunas and exercise to promote excretion of pesticide in sweat.

- **Observation**

  Review progress and send blood for serial pesticide levels.

- **Notification**

  Report case to your local Health and Safety Executive (see local phone book for number).

  Advise Pesticide Incidents Appraisal Panel of events.

The reason that detoxification works is that it reduces the total load of *all* pollutants. The threshold for symptoms in any individual will vary from day to day but provided that the 'total load' is below this level the patient will feel well (see Figure 3.7). Symptoms appear when the combined level of pollutants (D 'Total Level') exceeds the body's capacity to detoxify all these simultaneously. The body is able to tolerate either a level of pesticide (A) or car fumes (B) or food additives [E nos] (C) individually without obvious problems but together they cause symptoms.

Fertilizers (Nitrates)

Plants require nutrients from the soil before they can grow. One of the essential nutrients is nitrogen. Only a small proportion of the nitrogen in the soil is free (inorganic nitrogen NO_3) and available for plant growth. The rest is bound in decaying plants and animal

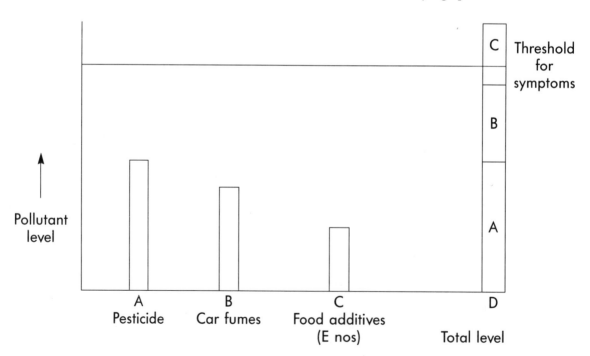

Figure 3.7 **'Total load' effect of pesticide with other pollutants**

manure. Plant growth can be accelerated dramatically by putting nitrate (NO_3) or ammonia (NH_3) fertilizer on the soil. However, only about half of the applied nitrate fertilizer is taken up by the growing plant. The other half is leached out by rain and surface water. After a long delay, up to 20 or 30 years, the fertilizer finds its way into drinking water. The present nitrate level in drinking water reflects the application of fertilizers a generation ago. The nitrate level in drinking water is likely to rise 2 to 3 times in the early part of the twenty-first century.

The nitrate in water is converted to nitrite by bacteria in the mouth. This causes several problems: nitrites combine with haemoglobin (the red pigment in blood), to form the blue pigment methaemoglobin. Babies are particularly vulnerable to this change, and nitrites can cause the 'Blue Baby Syndrome', which may be life-threatening. Nitrites also encourage the development of stomach cancer.

Pharmaceutical drugs

Pharmaceutical drugs that have powerful effects also have the capacity to produce powerful side-effects. Half the British population have slightly defective liver enzymes and are what is called 'slow acetylators' (i.e., their liver enzymes can only break down certain drugs slowly). Slow acetylators are more likely to suffer from drug-induced side effects, for example rashes. The very young and the old are also more likely to suffer from drug-induced side-effects. This is because their livers and other enzyme systems are less efficient than those of the young and middle-aged.

Iatrogenic diseases (diseases caused by doctors giving the wrong drug or too high a dose) are, unfortunately, very common (probably at least 1 in 10 of all illnesses). One of the first measures often tried when admitting a confused pensioner to hospital is to take him or her off all medication. A large proportion get dramatically better.

Drugs are made up of two parts: the active ingredient, and the base, which contains additives. Sometimes, the problem caused by a drug is not related to the active ingredient but to the base (the filler used to make up the weight), or the additives (colourings, flavourings and preservatives). Some allergic patients react to the lactose (milk sugar) or cornflour used as a base. Others react to the additives. Until recently, a well-known antihistamine tablet which was used to treat allergic conditions contained tartrazine (E102) which is a frequent cause of allergic reactions.

Dyes

Dyes are a major cause of allergies and sensitivities. By far the biggest source of the problems are azo food dye additives, which have no nutritional value but are used to 'improve' the appearance of food. Azo food dyes particularly affect individuals who are already allergic to aspirin. About one fifth of aspirin-sensitive people, most commonly middle-aged women, are also allergic to azo dyes.

Fabric dyes may also cause chemical sensitivities, especially aniline and chromate dyes. As a general rule, the lighter the dye, and the more natural the source, the less likely it is to cause problems.

Plastics

These synthetic substances affect chemically sensitive people due to 'outgassing' (i.e. release of gases, including formaldehyde and plasticizers). As a general rule, the harder the plastic, the less outgassing that occurs. Older plastics, like Bakelite and Formica, are usually safe. However, the modern *soft* plastics are much more likely to cause a problem. If you can mark them with your fingernail, or smell them, they are more likely to give you a problem. The worst plastics for outgassing are polythenes (plastic containers), polyvinyls (plastic curtains, upholstery and pipes), silicone seals, epoxy glues, polyurethane foams and stuffings, and teflon kitchen utensils.

Synthetic fibres and fabrics

Synthetic fibres and fabrics can cause allergies because they both release formaldehyde. If your chemical sensitivity is caused by synthetic fibres and fabrics, then you can remain in good health by dressing in natural fabrics, for example cotton and wool. (Check that the wool or cotton have not been treated with pesticides.) Large areas of synthetic fibres may also be found in curtains, carpets, upholstery, wall coverings and bed clothes. The worst fibres for outgassing formaldehyde are polyesters.

Soaps and detergents

Natural soap made without perfume is generally safe. However, modern detergents are manufactured from petrochemicals and may give problems. Especially bad are those 'biological' powders containing enzymes. After a machine wash there is quite enough detergent left in clothes to produce symptoms in susceptible individuals.

Skin irritation is the commonest problem caused by detergents. This tends to appear in the areas covered by clothes i.e. body and tops of limbs, and will generally be absent from hands and face. Skin irritation is a form of contact dermatitis. Detergents used for washing up dishes tend to cause contact dermatitis of the hands, especially in the webs between the fingers.

To avoid soap and detergent chemical sensitivity reduce your exposure to them in the following ways:

- When washing your body, use simple soap with no perfume;
- When washing clothes, a non-biological detergent should be used. There are now many ecologically safe detergents on the market which are also less likely to cause allergies;
- After you have washed your clothes with powder, put them through a further washing cycle *without any powder*.

Perfumes and cosmetics

Allergy to perfumes and cosmetics is a problem experienced almost exclusively by women. Some women are chemically sensitive both to their own and other womens' perfumes and cosmetics. If you find that you are sensitive to cosmetics, then there will often be enough in the air next to a wearer to give you a problem. It is wise to use low allergy cosmetics even if you have no chemical sensitivity, however, if you do have a problem you will need to avoid them completely.

Treated papers, boards and woods

Although these are all made from wood, they are impregnated with chemicals such as phenols, formaldehyde and occasionally the extremely poisonous dioxins. Laminated boards, block boards and plywoods are a major cause of indoor pollution in modern house construction, as they give off large amounts of formaldehyde.

Chlorinated hydrocarbons (the halocarbons)

The chlorine-carbon bond (Cl–C) found in chlorinated hydrocarbons has a particularly powerful effect on the immune system, stimulating it into response and often sensitivity. The chlorinated hydrocarbons are among the most toxic substances known. This is due to their persistence in the body fat, and, as 'orphan' chemicals, their almost complete resistance to being broken down.

This group includes:

organochlorine pesticides
PCBs (polychlorinated biphenyls)
solvents, polishes and cleaners
plasticizers
flame retardants
anaesthetics and pharmaceutical drugs
aerosol propellants (CFCs) and refrigerants

Chlorinated hydrocarbons are also produced during the chlorination of water, bleaching of paper and many other industrial processes. PCBs are very inert substances, which are excellent electric insulators but surprisingly good conductors of heat. For these properties they are used in transformers, electrical equipment and as hydraulic fluid.

CFCs, used as the propellant gas in aerosols are responsible for destruction of the ozone layer (see Chapter 4).

Toxic Gases

These include carbon monoxide, oxides of nitrogen, sulphur dioxide and ozone. The first two are produced by combusion of hydro-carbons e.g. petrol, diesel, natural gas. Sulphur dioxide is the main active ingredient in *acid rain*, which is responsible for the destruction of forests. Sulphur dioxide and oxides of nitrogen are produced by power stations burning sulphur-containing coal. The sulphur can be removed from the exhaust gases by the use of 'scrubbers'. Ozone (O_3) is produced by electrical devices, especially motors, and occurs due to poor contact and sparking. The 'ozone layer' surrounding the earth is *not* toxic, because it is situated 12 to 30 miles above the earth, and actually protects us against cosmic radiation.

Toxic Metals

These include the metals lead, mercury, cadmium and aluminium.

Lead

The main source of lead is as an anti-knocking agent in petrol. Lead also occurs in paint, lead pipes and joints, canned foods, juices and fruits. Fortunately, with the Green Awareness Campaign and the reduced price of lead-free petrol, the amount of this poison is dropping. Another source of lead is from food tins with unlined seams.

Lead is particularly destructive to children's brains. Studies have shown that high levels of lead found in children living near motorways cause a reduction in their IQ. Miscarriages and birth defects are also more common in areas with high lead levels.

Mercury

Mercury is one of the most toxic metals known. It is particularly poisonous when combined with other molecules to form organic mercury. In Japan, it is responsible for 'Minamata disease', caused by the pollution of tuna fish with industrial mercury.

The commonest source of mercury pollution is dental fillings. Mercury (a liquid metal) is used to produce amalgams of gold and silver which are used to make dental fillings. Research indicates that the mercury does not remain in the filling but is slowly leached out into the mouth from where it can be absorbed into the body. Mercury fillings have been implicated in a wide variety of diseases, including multiple sclerosis, epilepsy, psychiatric illnesses and ME. If amalgam fillings are removed in the correct order, i.e. the most dangerous one first, it is sometimes possible to cure these diseases. The dental cavities are, of course, refilled with a safe inert material.

Other common sources of mercury include:

- factories making paper;
- polluted drinking water;
- weed killers and mercury powders used to treat seed wheat;
- sea food from bottom of ocean;
- skin lightening creams.

Cadmium

The commonest source of cadmium is cigarette smoke. However, cadmium may occur in drinking water (due to its use in plumbing alloys), evaporated milk, shellfish and paints.

Arsenic

Arsenic is found in some insecticides, wines, well water, and shellfish, and is also produced by burning coal.

Aluminium

There are several common sources of aluminium. It most frequently occurs in tap water. Aluminium salts are added as a 'fining agent' during the purification process, in order to make biological matter such as weeds and algae drop out of suspension.

The metal also enters the body from aluminium cooking pots, pans, and foil, especially when cooking acid fruits such as rhubarb, apples and leaf vegetables. Aluminium pressure cookers give an even higher dose of the metal in the food. Aluminium teapots leach the metal into solution, and tea leaves have a particular ability to dissolve it. Aluminium is used to pack 'take away' foods, pre-packed frozen dinners and for some drinks cans. The metal is a component of certain foods and medicines, e.g. coffee creamers and some indigestion mixtures.

Alcohol

Alcohols are found in plastics, cleaning products, office solvents and drugs. Alcoholic beverages contain a particular sort of alcohol called ethyl alcohol (C_2H_5OH). Alcohol is a drug of addiction and is dealt with in further depth in Chapter 13. However, some people who react to alcohol are, in fact, allergic to the yeast used in the fermentation.

Ethyl alcohol drops given under the tongue can sometimes be used to desensitize a chemically sensitive patient to a wide variety of other chemicals.

Phenols

Phenol (carbolic acid) is a constituent of a very wide variety of household goods, including hard plastics (Bakelite), epoxy resins, phenolic resins, synthetic detergents, carbolic soap, disinfectants, dyes, preservatives, cosmetics and deodorants, pesticides and herbicides. It also occurs in the gold coloured lining of tin cans.

Terpenes

They are widely found in nature, especially in scented oils from pine trees and citrus fruits. Terpenes are found in the following synthetic sources: paints, motor car and gas fumes, and anaesthetics. The odour of terpenes is best described as the 'Christmas tree' smell.

Formaldehyde

Last but certainly not least, is formaldehyde. It is the single most important substance likely to induce chemical sensitivity. Approximately one person in five has a sensitivity to formaldehyde. It can cause symptoms at concentrations of as little as 1 part per 100 million. The symptoms are very varied, and include headaches, depression, fatigue, concentration and memory problems, dizziness, breathing problems, flushes and burnings, rashes, arthritis, flu like illness and changes in behaviour (all typical allergic symptoms).

Formaldehyde is outgassed (i.e. released as a gas) by a *very wide variety* of substances, including plastics, textiles, dyes, rubbers, foams, resins, glues, papers, newsprint, disinfectants, cosmetics, soaps, shampoos, insecticides, fertilizers, chipboard, block-board, plywood, veneer, concrete, plaster and motor car fumes, in fact, almost every synthetic item in the modern home.

Urea formaldehyde foam insulation (UFFI) is used in modern house insulation. It is put in the cavity wall and is made by mixing two chemicals which react together to form foam, the bubbles being produced by formaldehyde. UFFI continues to release formaldehyde into the house for many years after the insulation is installed, and can be a major cause of ill health. UFFI is banned in Canada. Other places which often have high formaldehyde levels include biology laboratories, shopping arcades, caravans, mobile houses and airtight houses and offices.

OUTDOOR AND INDOOR POLLUTION

It is helpful to divide chemical sensitivity into two groups on the basis of source:

- Outdoor pollution
- Indoor pollution.

The two usually have completely different causes. Although the treatment in both cases is avoidance, this is achieved in different ways.

What is likely to make my outdoor chemical sensitivity worse?

Outdoor pollution causing chemical sensitivity is usually intermittent rather than continuous. It can be predicted by the following factors:

- The amount of neotoxin released by the source, e.g. factory chimney, car fumes from underpasses, pesticide spray.
- How close you are to the source of neotoxins. For the technically minded, the amount of neotoxin you receive is usually proportional to the inverse square of the distance from the source: the amount received $= \dfrac{1}{d^2}$.
- The amount of time that you are exposed to the neotoxin. If you are sensitive to sulphur dioxide from a factory chimney, you may be able to drive past the factory without symptoms. However, if you live or work near the factory, then you will be constantly unwell.

The above three factors can be expressed in the formula which applies to all neotoxins (biological, chemical, physical and mental):

Dose of   = Amount of × 'proximity' × time
neotoxin   neotoxin   to source   exposed to
                                  of neotoxin   neotoxin

Other factors influencing reaction to outdoor pollutants are:

- *The wind direction.* Any location which is within 50 miles downwind of a large city is likely to suffer pollution. The wind usually blows from one direction (the prevailing wind), which means the areas downwind in the direction of the prevailing wind will be worst affected, whereas other areas will tend to be spared;
- *The wind strength.* Static air and winds above 15 miles per hour reduce the likelihood of chemical sensitivity whereas mild breezes increase the risk;
- *The humidity and cloud cover.* The more humid the atmosphere the more likely that an

airborne chemical will induce a chemical sensitivity. The most obvious example of this is fog, which, when mixed with a chemical pollutant, becomes smog. Exposure to smog for a day or two can induce a permanent sensitivity which will affect you for the rest of your life;

● *Geography of an area.* Some areas, e.g. Los Angeles (being located in a natural bowl-shaped area) tend to trap pollutants.

One useful way to assess the level of outdoor pollution is by measuring visibility. As a general rule, the greater the distance you can see, the less the level of outdoor pollution.

Which sort of pollution is more likely to cause my chemical sensitivity, outdoor or indoor?

Superficially, it would appear that outdoor pollution is a more serious problem than indoor pollution. However, in practice, the opposite is the case. Indoor pollution causes chemical sensitivity in 8 to 10 times as many people as outdoor pollution. This is why your chemical sensitivity is likely to be better outdoors, and in the summer, and worse indoors and in the winter, when ventilation is reduced and the central heating is on.

Which factors make indoor pollution worse?

Modern construction methods

These usually involve the use of materials that outgas formaldehyde and other organic fumes. These materials include chipboard, block-board, particle board, treated timbers and plywood, plastics, solvents, glues, paints, varnishes, pesticides and fungicides.

Modern furnishing methods

Extensive use of synthetic fabrics, carpets and plastics produces a large 'load' of formaldehyde and other gases.

Lack of ventilation

Many modern buildings have airtight seals on the windows and are designed to have little or no outside ventilation. In large buildings, air conditioning and ventilation systems recirculate indoor air without removing the formaldehyde and other gases. Consequently, the air 'purification' system tends to concentrate gases that may induce chemical sensitivities.

The heating system/kitchen

These may be the origin of fumes that induce chemical sensitivity.

Cleaning substances

Wide use of cleaners, polishes, solvents, aerosols, air fresheners and disinfectants.

Integral garages and storerooms

These allow vehicle combustion fumes and other solvent fumes to enter working and living areas.

Wide use of plastic-covered electronic devices

Apart from the electric and magnetic fields which are deal with in Chapter 4, these cause problems because they get hot and release chemical fumes and ozone, e.g. television sets, photocopying machines, and power tools.

Biological neotoxins

These are not chemical neotoxins. However, they contribute to the total load of neotoxins in the house. These include house dust mites (minute insects living in bedding, carpets and curtains), pollen (from house plants and other indoor vegetation), cats' and other domestic animals' fur, fungi (from damp areas, especially bathrooms, basements and under sinks).

How can I remove particulate air pollution?

Particulate air pollution can be removed in three basic ways:

Mechanical air filter
Ionizer and electrostatic cleaner
Activated carbon filter.

The method depends on the particle size that you wish to remove. The following table gives an indication of cleaning methods suitable for each particle size.

How do I find out to which chemicals I am sensitive?

This is rather similar to the food exclusion method and consists of five stages: suspicion, pretesting, exclusion, challenge and load reduction.

Suspicion

Suspect chemical sensitivity if you have any of the diseases listed on page 65. The symptoms of which are most likely to be caused by chemicals are ones affecting the brain, including fatigue, reduced concentration and memory, feeling 'doped up', irritability, excitability, and feeling 'high'. Chemical sensitivity is greatly underdiagnosed. If you don't suspect it, you can't find it. Discovery depends upon the prepared mind.

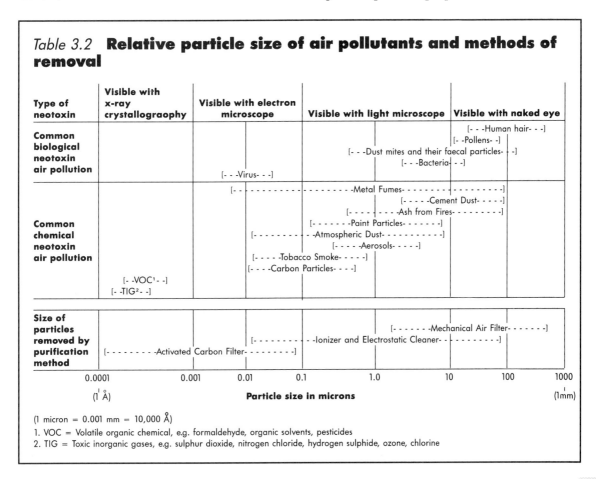

Table 3.2 **Relative particle size of air pollutants and methods of removal**

Type of neotoxin	Visible with x-ray crystallograophy	Visible with electron microscope	Visible with light microscope	Visible with naked eye
Common biological neotoxin air pollution		[- - -Virus- - -]	[- - -Dust mites and their faecal particles- - -] [- - -Bacteria- - -]	[- - -Human hair- - -] [- -Pollens- -]
Common chemical neotoxin air pollution	[- -VOC¹- -] [- -TIG²- -]	[- - - - - - - - - Atmospheric Dust- - - - - - - - - -] [- - - -Tobacco Smoke- - - - -] [- - - -Carbon Particles- - - -]	[- - - - - - - - - - - - - -Metal Fumes- - - - - - - - - - - - - - -] [- - - - - - - -Ash from Fires- - - - - - - -] [- - - - - -Paint Particles- - - - - -] [- - - -Aerosols- - - -]	[- - - -Cement Dust- - - -]
Size of particles removed by purification method	[- - - - - - - -Activated Carbon Filter- - - - - - - -]	[- - - - - - - - - -Ionizer and Electrostatic Cleaner- - - - - - - - - -]		[- - - - - -Mechanical Air Filter- - - - - -]

0.0001	0.001	0.01	0.1	1.0	10	100	1000
(1 Å)				Particle size in microns			(1mm)

(1 micron = 0.001 mm = 10,000 Å)
1. VOC = Volatile organic chemical, e.g. formaldehyde, organic solvents, pesticides
2. TIG = Toxic inorganic gases, e.g. sulphur dioxide, nitrogen chloride, hydrogen sulphide, ozone, chlorine

Pretesting and recording of symptoms, places and activities

Before you start testing for chemical sensitivities, you must first make sure you don't have food allergies. To identify a food allergy follow the method as described in Chapter 2. Make sure you are eating an organic diet which is completely free of chemicals and pesticides. Also give up smoking or reduce your consumption as much as possible. Smoking is a massive cause of internal chemical pollution.

Chemical sensitivity tends to come and go more quickly than food allergies. Food remains in the bowel for up to 3 days, whereas chemicals are absorbed rapidly through the lungs and excreted at a similar rate.

Fill in the chemical neotoxin diary (see page 87) for a week. Write down your symptoms, together with your activities and the places you have visited. Try to link your symptoms with the activities or places that caused them. Score your symptoms 0 to 4 using the following scoring system:

```
0 = no symptoms
1 = very mild symptoms
2 = moderate symptoms
3 = severe symptoms
4 = very severe symptoms
```

Weigh yourself naked first thing in the morning (after emptying your bladder and if possible, opening your bowels) and last thing at night.

Use the method of pulse testing. Take your pulse every hour. Make sure you have been sitting still for 2 minutes before testing and have not exerted yourself violently with the preceding 5 minutes.

Use the Handwriting Test at the bottom of the Chemical Neotoxin Diary. Copy the standard sentence, 'The quick brown fox jumps over the lazy dog' when you are feeling well. Then copy it again if you think you have had a reaction to a chemical. If you have had a genuine reaction you will probably notice a drastic deterioration in the quality of your writing.

By the end of the pretesting period you are likely to have had some symptoms. The diary will allow you to link the symptoms with an activity or place. It is not practical to test yourself with hundreds of chemicals. This pretesting stage enables you to narrow down the likely culprits.

Excluding chemical neotoxins

It usually takes 4 to 24 hours to clear your body of chemical neotoxins. However, to make sure you are not suffering from the 'masking' effect, try to reduce your exposure to all chemicals for 4 days. The 'masking' effect is described in greater depth on page 33.

You may initially feel worse when the chemical to which you are sensitive is removed (unmasking causes a hangover). You may then feel better when the chemical is returned (masking). However, if you stay away from the substance to which you are chemically sensitive for more than 3 days, the masking effect disappears.

You can assist the clearance of chemical neotoxins by the following methods:

1. Go to an unpolluted spot and take five very deep breaths. Have a couple of minutes rest and repeat. The deep breathing will encourage excretion of chemicals that have built up in your body.
2. Exercise enough to make you sweat. Neotoxins are excreted in sweat. This excretion can be assisted by taking a sauna, which artificially makes you sweat.
3. Stay out of the house and car all day. Travel by foot or bicycle and avoid polluted areas.
4. Turn your bedroom into a low allergy haven, as described on page 145.

Table 3.3 **Chemical neotoxin diary**

Name..................... Day........... Date........... Weight naked...........am...........
pm...........

Time	Description of Symptoms	Rate Symptoms 0–4	Pulse Rate	Activity	Place	Comments
06.00						
08.00						
10.00						
12.00						
14.00						
16.00						
18.00						
20.00						
22.00						
24.00						
02.00						
04.00						

Scoring system
0 = no symptoms
1 = mild symptoms
2 = moderate symptoms
3 = severe symptoms
4 = very severe symptoms

Pulse Rate: Count your pulse rate every hour and write it down in bpm in the column marked 'Pulse Rate'

Hand writing test
Test: 'The quick brown fox jumps over the lazy dog'   Time   Date

....
....
....

At the end of this exclusion period you should be feeling much better. You will then be able to start testing. During this time you may notice that your sense of smell returns, or even becomes very acute.

Challenge

You will need the help of a friend or family member for the challenge stage, which is best carried out in the open air. The pretesting stage should have given you an inkling of which chemical(s) may be causing your problem. For example, you may find that you are worse when you are in your kitchen or returning to work on a Monday. Make a note of all the things in the kitchen or at work that could be affecting you.

When you are feeling well, challenge yourself with likely chemicals between meals. The way you do this is to get your assistant to prepare several air tight jam jars filled with traces of the substance to which you think you

---

Table 3.4 **Challenge Diary**

Name............................. Day............... Date............... Pulse rate resting...............

Chemical Tested	Symptoms	Score symptoms 0–4	Pulse Rate	Comments

0 = no symptoms
1 = very mild symptoms
2 = moderate symptoms
3 = severe symptoms
4 = very severe symptoms

may be chemically sensitive.

If you think that you might be allergic to polyester fibres, your assistant should put a square of material in a jam jar for three days and use it to test you. Fumes can be collected from other sources by leaving a jam jar open for half an hour next to likely sources of chemical sensitivity, e.g. photocopying machines, gas cookers.

Test yourself by putting the jar two feet away from your face and take a few deep breaths. Keep the jar open for 20 minutes and look for a reaction. Symptoms of reaction include headache, dizziness, nausea, irritability, depression, palpitations or a pulse rate change of more than 20 beats per minute. *DO NOT TEST YOURSELF WITH HIGHLY POISONOUS SUBSTANCES LIKE PESTICIDES.*

Write down your reactions in the challenge diary (page 88). First, test chemicals to which you are unlikely to be allergic. Keep the most likely candidates to which you think you might be allergic until last. You are likely to be allergic to chemicals whose smell you are particularly fond of.

If you have a reaction:

- remove the chemical;
- take some deep breaths of clear air;
- take one teaspoonful of sodium bicarbonate in a glass of spring water. This helps to neutralize the reaction by making your body less acidic;
- stop testing for that day.

Long-term chemical load reduction

Having identified your chemical neotoxin(s) (there may be more than one), there are a few things that you must do to maintain health:

1. Completely avoid or greatly reduce the exposure to the chemicals to which you are particularly sensitive;
2. Reduce your total load of neotoxins (see Chapter 6).
3. Use sleep and rest, exercise, vitamins, minerals and other supplements to help yourself back to complete health.

SUMMARY

- Chemical pollution is now alarmingly widespread and all over the world. We are reaching, (or have passed) the planet's capacity to recycle all the chemicals that are being produced.
- Chemical allergies are more accurately called sensitivities and usually begin because of excessive exposure to a single chemical. If the body is constantly exposed to that single chemical then cross-sensitivity to many chemicals is likely to develop.
- Chemical sensitivities can be triggered either by acute massive exposure or by chronic exposure.

- Chemicals are able to induce the general adaption syndrome with the recognized stages of alarm, adaption or resistance, and exhaustion.
- The commonest symptoms produced by chemicals are those that affect the brain, e.g. headache, irritability, tiredness, doped feeling.
- Symptoms caused by chemical sensitivity usually have a rapid onset.
- Chemicals enter the body by three routes: being eaten, inhaled or contact with the skin.
- Chemicals, especially fat soluble ones, tend to become bioconcentrated along

food chains. As humans are always at the end of the food chain they often receive high loads of chemicals in food.

● Tap water is commonly polluted with substances that may cause chemical sensitivity.

● Indoor pollution causes considerably more chemical sensitivity than outdoor pollution.

● The dose of neotoxin can be expressed by the formula:

$$\text{Dose of neotoxin} = \text{Amount of neotoxin at source} \times \text{proximity to source of neotoxin} \times \text{time exposed to neotoxin}$$

● You are likly to be able to find your own chemical neotoxin by first suspecting a chemical sensitivity and then correlating your symptoms with activities and places. To test for a chemical sensitivity challenge yourself with the likely chemical culprits provided that they are not actively poisonous, e.g. pesticides.

● Ways to beat chemical neotoxins:

1. Completely avoid or greatly reduce the exposure to the chemical(s) to which you are particularly sensitive

2. Reduce your total load of neotoxins.

3. Use sleep and rest, exercise, vitamins, minerals and other supplements to help yourself back to complete health.

CHAPTER FOUR

THE PHYSICAL NEOTOXINS: ELECTROMAGNETIC RADIATION, SOUND AND GEOPATHIC STRESS

One hundred years ago there were no domestic electrical devices. A century later in the western world it is impossible to find people who do not live and work in an 'electric smog'.

'Allergy' or electrical sensitivities can be caused by radiowaves, microwaves, light, ultra-violet (UV) rays, x-rays and sound. These neotoxins obey the laws of physics rather than chemistry, hence their classification as physical neotoxins. However, they are able to show all the features of chemical neotoxins such as masking, adaption, stimulation and the depression of the immune system, and the provocation/neutralization response.

The true significance of physics and electromagnetic waves has been greatly under-appreciated. Up until the present they have been used almost solely for diagnosis (x-rays, ultrasound, radioisotope, CAT and NMR scans). They are rarely used for treatment, though acupuncture and homoeopathy probably work due to their electromagnetic effect.

Medical treatments of the future will be based on a completely new way of treating people using the largely unexplored subject of medical physics. With research and development, there is little doubt that not just a whole new chapter, but a whole new library will be written of new cures for old diseases. These treatments will include identifying frequencies that are harmful to the body and screening these, and replacing them with other frequencies that promote health. On a very limited scale this has already been used to help patients with electrical sensitivity.

One of the shortcomings of conventional medicine is that doctors are still looking for chemical explanations for problems that are based in physics. To give an example: when the correct homoeopathic remedy is put under the tongue, a major improvement can occur in 1 to 2 seconds. This improvement is far too fast to be caused by a chemical reaction. The circulation time from mouth to the brain is at least 15 seconds. However, an alternative theory based on principles of physics could explain such a speed of reaction.

A further example is the unexplained communication that sometimes occurs between two people. This is unlikely to be due to chemistry because the speed of reaction and separation. However, an explanation based on physics in which one individual radiates a signal and the other receives it, though not proven, has a better chance of describing the observed events.

WHAT ARE THE SOURCES OF PHYSICAL NEOTOXINS?

Non-ionizing radiation ⎫ Electromagnetic
Ionizing radiation ⎬ radiation

Sound
Geopathic stress

WHAT IS THE SPECTRUM OF ELECTROMAGNETIC RADIATION?

Radiowaves, microwaves, light, UV and x-rays are all part of the electromagnetic spectrum (see Table 4.1). They are all waves, with differing wavelengths.

Wavelengths and frequency are related by the formula:

$$\text{Wavelength (in metres)} = \frac{\text{speed of light (in metres per second)}}{\text{frequency (in cycles per second)}}$$

For example: to find the wavelength of a 50 Hz (mains frequency) electrical current:

$$\text{Wavelength} = \frac{300,000,000\text{m}}{50\text{cps}} \quad \begin{aligned} &= 6,000,000\text{m} \\ &= 6,000\ \text{km} \end{aligned}$$

Thus the wavelength arising from a 50 Hz high voltage power line is 6,000 km i.e. from London to Nairobi.

Table 4.1 shows the electromagnetic spectrum. ELF waves (extra long frequency waves with wavelengths up to 10,000 km and longer). Start at the beginning of the table and work through to cosmic rays, which have wavelengths of $10 - {}^{15}$m.

● Electrical devices use 50 Hz (60 Hz in USA) with a wavelength of 6,000 km (5,000 km).
● Radio broadcasts use wavelengths of 10 km to 10 m.
● VHF radio, TV and telecommunications, and microwave and radar devices use wavelengths of 10m to 1mm.
● Ultra-violet, x-rays and gamma rays have even shorter wavelengths.

Table 4.1 **Electromagnetic spectrum and sources of electromagnetic radiation (non-ionizing radiation)**

Radio wave band (decreasing)	Frequency description (increasing)	Frequency (Hz)	Wavelength (in metres)	Sources and devices producing frequency
		3 Hz	10^7	
	ELF (Extremely Low Frequency			Power lines, and stations, EL blankets, hair dryers, soldering irons, electric trains and motors, VDU's
		3×10^2Hz	10^6	
Very Long	ULF Ultra Low Frequency)			Harmonics from HV power lines (300Hz) ? navy transmitters (very secret)
		3×10^3Hz	10^5	
	VLF (Very Low Frequency)			VDU's, coastal radiotelegraphy and marine radio beacons, induction systems
Long		3×10^4Hz	10^4	
	LF (Long Frequency)			Long wave AM radio, coastal radiotelegraphy, pagers, induction HTG systems, radio beacons
Medium		3×10^5Hz	10^3	
	MF (Medium Frequency)			Medium wave AM radio, radio beacons, cordless phones, radio distress signals
Short		3×10^6Hz	10^2	
	HF (High Frequency)			Short wave AM radio/radio hams, CB's including hearing aids
Ultra Short		3×10^7Hz	10	
	VHF (Very High Frequency)			FM radio, pagers, elderly alarm systems, radio phones and microphones, model planes, emergency services
		3×10^8Hz	1	
Microwave Band				
		3×10^8Hz	1	

Radio wave band (decreasing)	Frequency description (increasing)	Frequency (Hz)	Wavelength (in metres)	Sources and devices producing frequency
Decimetres	UHF (Ultra High Frequency)			TV, VDUs, pagers, rescue beacons, antitheft devices, cellular phones, CB's, satellite transmissions, marine radar, microwave ovens
		3×10^9Hz	10^{-1}	
Centimetres	SHF (Super High Frequency)			Airborne radar, doppler radar, space links, pagers, radio beacons
		3×10^{10}Hz	10^{-2}	
Millimetres	EHF (Extremely High Frequency)			High definition radar, satellite links
		3×10^{11}Hz	10^{-3}	
Infra Red	Infra Red Frequency			Sun, VDUs, night vision equipment and all hot bodies
		3×10^{14}Hz	10^{-6}	
Visible Light	Visible Light Frequency			Sun, VDU, fluorescent and filament lamps and hot bodies, lasers
		7.5×10^{14}Hz	4×10^{-7}	
	To Ultra Violet Light (Ionizing Radiation)			

Description of Waveband (Wavelength decreasing)	Frequency (Hz)	Wavelength (in metres)	Sources and devices producing frequency
(Visible Light (Non-Ionizing))			
(Ionizing Radiation)			

Description of Waveband (Wavelength decreasing)	Frequency (Hz)	Wavelength (in metres)	Sources and devices producing frequency
	7.5×10^{14}	4.0×10^{-7}	
Ultra Violet A			Sun and sun bed, VDU's
	9.4×10^{14}	3.2×10^{-7}	
Ultra Violet B			Sun – increased by depleted ozone layer
	1.1×10^{15}	2.8×10^{-7}	
Ultra Violet C			Sun – increased by depleted ozone layer
	1.5×10^{15}	2.0×10^{-7}	
X-rays			TV, VDU's, medical x-rays and radiotherapy
	3×10^{21}	10^{-11}	
Gamma Rays			Nuclear power stations and reprocessing plants, atom bombs and military bases, air travel
	3×10^{19}	10^{-13}	
Cosmic Rays			High levels found in space, air travel
	3×10^{23}	10^{-15}	

Table to show powers of Ten and prefixes

Power of Ten	Prefixes	Symbol
10^{18}	exa	E
10^{15}	peta	P
10^{12}	tera	T
10^9	giga	G
10^6	mega	M
10^3	kilo	k
10^2	hecto	h
10^1	deca	da
10^{-1}	deci	d
10^{-2}	centi	c
10^{-3}	milli	m

Conversion table from metres to other metric units of length

Metres		Other units
10^{12}m	=	1,000,000,000 Km
10^9m	=	1,000,000 Km
10^6m	=	1,000 Km
10^3m	=	1 Km
10^2m	=	100 m
10^1m	=	10 m
10^{-1}m	=	10 cm
10^{-2}m	=	1 cm
10^{-3}m	=	1 mm
10^{-6}m	=	1 micron
10^{-9}m	=	10 A°

Power of Ten	Prefixes	Symbol
10^{-6}	micro	μ
10^{-9}	nano	n
10^{-12}	pico	p
10^{-15}	femto	f
10^{-18}	atto	a

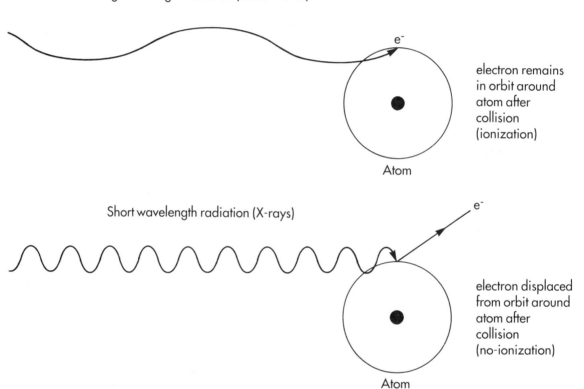

Figure 4.1 **The difference between non-ionizing and ionizing radiation**

WHAT IS THE DIFFERENCE BETWEEN NON-IONIZING AND IONIZING RADIATION?

The electromagnetic spectrum is further divided into non-ionizing radiation (NIR wavelength longer than 4×10^{-7}m), and ionizing radiation (IR Wavelength of shorter than 4×10^{-7}m). Ionizing radiation has a higher energy level than non-ionizing radiation. This higher energy level enables the ionizing radiation to knock an electron off an atom or molecule it collides with. This removal of the electron causes the atom to become charged or ionized, hence the name. See Figure 4.1.

It was realized a long time ago that ionizing radiation was dangerous. It can cause gene mutation and cancer. More recently, it has been realized that non-ionizing radiation is also dangerous, and that the two sorts of radiation have an additive effect.

HOW CAN I WORK OUT MY RISK OF EM RADIATION DAMAGE?

The dose of EM radiation can be worked out by using a formula which applies to all neotoxins:

Dose of EM = strength of × 'proximity' to × time
radiation   source (amount   source of   exposed to
                of neotoxin at   neotoxin   neotoxin
                source)

The biological effect is given by:

Biological effect of = Dose of   × Individual susceptibility
EM radiation   Neotoxin   (genetic and acquired
                                    factors)

Individual   = Genetic Influences × Acquired
Susceptibility   environmental
                                        influences

This formula will help you to predict whether you are likely to suffer the biological effect of EM radiation. To give you an example: if there is a high voltage power line (high strength source), and you live within 50 yards (close proximity to source), and you are in your house for 16 hours a day (long exposure), then your dose of physical neotoxin is high. In addition, if your individual susceptibility is high because your genes have given you a greater than usual susceptibility (genetic factors), and if your general state of health is poor and your total load of neotoxins is high (both acquired factors), then under these conditions the high voltage power line is very likely to make you ill.

IS THE HIGH VOLTAGE POWER LINE REALLY A HEALTH HAZARD?

There are several reasons why you may fail to realize that a physical neotoxin (e.g. electric and magnetic fields from a high voltage power line), is making you ill:

● The high voltage power line may initially stimulate you and make you feel better;
● If you move away from the high power voltage line within a short time, (e.g. 3 years), there may be no obvious effect;
● There is a long latent period (5 to 15 years) before a well defined disease shows itself. Up until that time the allergic problem tends to produce many poorly defined symptoms.

The following statistics should make doubters reconsider the evidence that electromagnetic waves are at present potential sources of disease.

● Cancers in electrical workers tend to occur 10 years earlier than the time that type of growth would usually be expected to occur.
● People working in high electric fields have between 3 and 13 times the usual incidence of brain tumours.
● Radio hams have a high incidence of leukaemias and other blood cancers.
● The incidence of childhood leukaemias around nuclear reprocessing plants is between 6 and 10 times the predicted level.

WHAT IS THE RELATIONSHIP BETWEEN ELECTROMAGNETIC WAVES, ELECTRIC FIELDS, MAGNETIC FIELDS AND RADIATION?

The effect of electromagnetic waves on the body is due to electric fields, magnetic fields and radiation. These are created as follows: An electric field is created by an electric voltage. The purest example of an electric field is static electricity which makes the hairs on the back of your hand stand up. The strength of the electric field is measured in volts per meter (v/m) and is proportional to the size of the voltage. Electric fields fall off rapidly from the source. (For the technically minded, the electric field at very long wavelengths is proportional to the inverse cube of the distance from the source. At shorter wavelengths the field is proportional to the inverse square of the distance from the source).

Magnetic fields are caused by magnets, and also by electric currents moving in conductors, for example an electromagnet used to pick up scrap iron in a junkyard or around an electric motor transformer. The strength of a magnetic field is measured in tesla, the earth's magnetic field being equivalent to approximately 50 microtesla. The magnetic field is dependent on the current flowing through the conductor. In comparison with electric fields, magnetic fields fall off more slowly with distance. (For the technically minded, they are proportional to the inverse square of the distance or sometimes even just to the inverse of the distance). Consequently, magnetic fields are more likely to cause illness than electric fields.

Radiation is given off by radioactive materials, and also when an electric charge is accelerated or decelerated, as, for example, in a fluorescent tube, when light is produced because the electric field causes charged atoms to accelerate along the tube.

CAN ELECTRIC FIELDS, MAGNETIC FIELDS AND RADIATION BE SCREENED FROM THE BODY?

Electrical fields can be screened from the body fairly easily by using what is called Gaussian screening or a Faraday cage. It has been found that if an object is completely covered with an earthed metal foil or wire cage, then it will completely shield the enclosed object. This useful effect is used to screen co-axial cable, which carries television signals from the aerial to the television set.

Magnetic fields are much more difficult to screen. Iron and other metal alloys (mumetal) are known to attract magnetic fields, which then run through the screening metal rather than through objects inside the screen. However, it is very difficult to completely screen an object from magnetic fields.

Radiation consists of three different types:

alpha	}	These are produced by decay of radioactive elements and can be screened by cardboard or
beta		water.
gamma	–	No material stops these rays completely but they are greatly attenuated (reduced) by feet of concrete or lead.

Successful screening reduces the three factors mentioned in the neotoxin dose equation on page 95:

- The strength or *amount* of radiation is reduced by the lead or other screen;
- The proximity to *source* is reduced by being far enough away from the source;
- The *time* of exposure is reduced by moving away from the radiation.

WHAT FACTORS AFFECT ELECTRICAL SENSITIVITY?

Food allergy and chemical sensitivity affect about half the population. Some of these allergic people also become electrically sensitive (at least 1 in 1,000 of the population on present estimates). These electrically sensitive people often radiate a weak electromagnetic field themselves when they are reacting allergically. This radiation can affect electronic equipment (e.g. computers, washing machines, car ignitions), and stop them from working properly.

The features of an electromagnetic wave that decide whether it will affect an electrically sensitive person are frequency, coherence, wave form and intensity.

Frequency

An electrically sensitive person may react to several different frequencies, from ELF to microwave frequencies.

Coherence

A coherent wave is a very pure wave of just one frequency (like playing a single note on the piano). In nature most EM waves, e.g. sunlight, are not at all coherent (like playing all the notes on the piano softly at once). Consequently, the non-coherent waves, common in nature, are far less likely to trigger an allergic reaction. Man-made waves, in contrast, are much more coherent, and certain frequencies keep recurring as they come from many different sources, for example the 50 cycles mains frequency.

The body uses many extra low frequencies itself (see Table 4.2). When the body is exposed to a large number of man-made ELF frequencies, the immune system becomes overloaded and starts to give symptoms. Some forms of man-made EM waves are completely coherent. A laser (Light Application by Stimulated Emission of Radiation) produces only a very narrow waveband, consisting of one frequency alone.

Waveform

In nature, most waves are sinusoidal in shape (like an 'S' on its side). However, pulsed waves (which are saw toothed or square and are usually man-made) have a far greater ability to penetrate cells and cause damage. Pulsed waves are very similar to the waves produced by a nerve cell when it sends an electrical message to the brain.

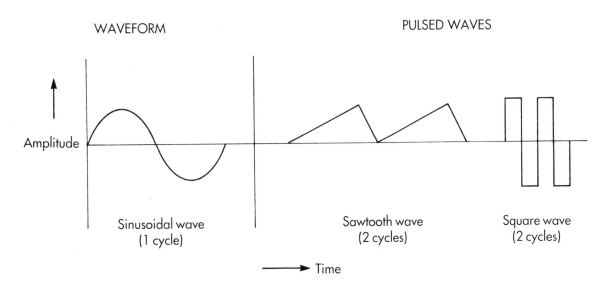

Figure 4.2 **Different types of waveform**

Table 4.2 Important electromagnetic frequencies affecting the body

Frequency in Hz (cycles per sec)	Description of frequency/therapy	System/organ affected by frequency	Comment
1–2 Hz	Heartbeat	Heart	ECG shows electrical health of heart and is invaluable for diagnosis
1.5–4 Hz	Delta Rhythm	Brain	An EEG (electroencephalograph) shows the electrical health of the brain
4–7 Hz	Theta Rhythm		Delta rhythm = not normally found in adults Theta rhythm = found near temples in normal subjects
8–13 Hz	Alpha Rhythm		Alpha rhythm = meditation frequency: disappears with eyes open – intellectual activity
18–30 Hz	Beta Rhythm		Beta rhythm = associated with anxiety
100–1500 Hz	Electrosleep and electroanaesthesia	Brain	Small currents at these frequencies can be used by trained practitioner to induce sleep and remove pain
25 or 40 Hz	Electro convulsive therapy (ECT)	Brain	Used to induce fit to treat severe depression
5 Hz	Interferential Therapy	Brain	Alters mood and induces depression
8–10 Hz			Alters mood and induces well-being
0–5 Hz	An ELF current is produced by the difference between two higher frequencies (the 'beat' frequency)	Autonomic nervous system (controls unconscious functions, eg, breathing, bowels, pupils, sweating and blood pressure)	Stimulates sympathetic nerves (greater level of excitement)
10–15 Hz			Stimulates parasympathetic nerves (lower level of excitement)
10–15 Hz		Nerve fibres	Stimulates nerves that control movements
90–110 Hz			Stimulates sensory nerves that perceive touch
130 Hz			Stimulate pain fibres
0–10 Hz		Smooth muscle (as found in heart, bowel, bronchi and uterus)	Stimulate smooth muscle to constrict
15–200 Hz	Transcutaneous nerve stimulation	Peripheral nerve	Used for pain relief
27.5, 55, 110, 220, 440, 880 Hz	Electrotherapy	Whole body	27.5 and its even harmonics (i.e. 55 = 27.5×2 110 = 27.5×4)
10^{-3} Hz	Acupuncture	Whole body	Works along meridians. Each organ/system has its own meridian along the body and electric voltages can be detected at acupuncture points. These change with disease
Varies with remedy and potency	Homoeopathy	Whole body	Homoeopathic tablet contains healing frequency, specific for each remedy
2 MHz–2.45 Gh	Electrocautery and diathermy/shortwave and microwave	Whole body	Used in surgery to cauterize and cut tissues without stimulating nerve or muscle
1–10 GH	DNA resonant frequency	Cell nucleus	At selected frequencies in this range DNA molecules vibrate
1–30 Hz (especially 7, 14 and 21 Hz	Schumann waves	Whole body	Produced by thunderstorms setting earth and ionosphere into resonance like a giant 'electrical' bell

There are electrical components in television sets that produce electrical and magnetic pulse waves. Consequently, television sets and VDUs are common sources of this waveform.

Intensity

Rather surprisingly, the intensity of a wave is far less important than its frequency, coherence and waveform. Providing that the intensity of a wave is greater than the threshold (which can be very low), it will cause an electrical sensitivity. The threshold for sensitivity to a 50 Hz magnetic field can be as low as 30 nanotesla (nanotesla = 10^{-9} tesla); earth's magnetic field is 50 microtesla but static (microtesla = 10^{-6} tesla).

HOW CAN I TELL IF I AM ELECTRICALLY SENSITIVE?

Almost all electrically sensitive people are also sufferers from food and/or chemical allergies. There are a number of other common findings that often occur in electrically sensitive people:

- electrical equipment often malfunctions, e.g. computers, washing machines, electric car ignitions, won't operate normally;
- quartz watches do not work when you wear them;
- you may frequently get electric shocks from objects, especially cars, that do not affect other people;
- you are unable to wear synthetic fibres, especially nylon, due to the build up of static electricity;
- 'earthing' yourself is often helpful. This consists of walking barefoot on the grass or on concrete for half an hour a day;
- fluorescent lighting may make you feel unwell. However, full spectrum fluorescent lights are much less of a problem;

- water often has a positive effect and you feel much better near rivers, lakes and seas. Taking a bath or shower also improves your condition providing that the water has not been exposed to an electrical frequency that gives you problems;
- you feel worse before a thunderstorm.

Symptoms of electrical sensitivity include all the allergic symptoms mentioned in Chapter 1. However, those particularly associated with electric and magnetic fields include flushing and blushing, palpitations, diarrhoea, muscular aches, noises in the head, pins and needles, especially in hands and feet, dizziness, fits and blackouts, disorientation, headaches, depression and persistent tiredness unrelieved by rest. Electrical sensitivity may also mimic neurological diseases such as paralysis, epilepsy and MS.

Electrical provocation-neutralization testing may be used to test for electrical sensitivity in a similar way to provocation-neutralization testing for food and chemical allergies. Instead of injecting extracts under the skin or placing them under the tongue, the patient is tested with EM waves produced from a frequency generator.

In an electrically sensitive person:

- One frequency will provoke symptoms and another frequency will neutralize (remove) them;
- The strength of the signal is unimportant provided that it is greater than the threshold;
- The frequency provoking symptoms is usually specific for each patient and that frequency has no effect on a non-electrically sensitive person (the tester).

HOW CAN I BE TREATED IF I AM AN ELECTRICALLY SENSITIVE PERSON?

Once the best neutralization frequency has been located it is possible to 'store' this frequency either in a glass vial of water or in a homoeopathic tablet of the correct remedy and potency. The glass vial is prepared, by placing it in a coil of wire energized at the neutralizing frequency. This glass vial will then help the electrically sensitive patient to feel better for up to two months.

WHY DOES AN ELECTRICALLY SENSITIVE PERSON BECOME SO REACTIVE TO THE WRONG EM FREQUENCY?

An electrically sensitive person is often exquisitely sensitive to the wrong EM frequency. This exquisite sensitivity is caused by the body's remarkable ability to react to the smallest possible packet of energy (a quantum or, in the case of light, a photon).

In order to understand this incredible sensitivity it is helpful to look at the way that the normal eye functions. When your eye is 'dark adapted', you will first be able to see a single photon light energy reaching the retina. The amount of energy contained in this photon is incredibly small. However, the amount of energy required to stimulate a nerve fibre to send a message to the brain is far, far larger (1 millivolt which is about 10^{10} times more energy than has arrived in a single photon). Fortunately, there is a very high amplification system in the retina cell which gives a gain of the order to 10^{10} as shown in Figure 4.3.

Allergy or electrical sensitivity occurs when the enzyme system becomes constantly switched on and keeps sending messages to the

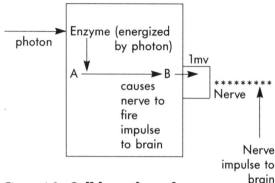

Figure 4.3 **Cell in retina of eye**

brain as if light were being continually received by the retina.

WHY ARE EXTRA LOW FREQUENCIES (ELF WAVES, 0 TO 300 HZ) A PARTICULAR HEALTH HAZARD TO THE BODY?

As you will see from Figure 4.3 above, the body uses many low frequencies for its own purposes. The heartbeat is 1 to 2 Hz, the brain waves are from 1–20 Hz. Other frequencies in the ELF band are used by therapists to stimulate the body, especially the brain and nervous system. Frequencies used for electrocautery and diathermy are particularly chosen so that they will be considerably higher than those used in the body. Consequently, they do not stimulate nerves to conduct a message or muscles to contract.

Nature produces frequencies in the ELF range called Schumann waves. Schumann waves have frequencies in the range 1 Hz to 30 Hz, and most commonly occur at the harmonies 7, 14, and 21 Hz. They are produced because the earth itself, and ionosphere (60 km above the earth's surface), act as a giant electrical resonator. This resonace is energized by thunderstorms. At any moment in time there are about 2,000 thunderstorms occurring around the world. The thunderstorms themselves, create frequencies of 0.001 Hz to 20 kHz. Part of the reason that some people are so adversely affected by weather is because of the ELF waves produced.

WHAT IS THE RELATIONSHIP BETWEEN SOUND WAVES AND ELECTROMAGNETIC WAVES?

It is a surprising finding that electromagnetic and sound waves are interchangeable in plant and animal cells. This interchangeability occurs because of an interesting property of the cell membrane which acts in a way similar to a piezo-electric crystal in a gramophone needle. A typical cell is 1,000th to 1 tenth of a millimetre long. However, the cell membrane is only 1/100,000th of a millimetre thick (10^{-8} m). There is an electric drop (voltage) of 1 tenth of a volt across the cell membrane from outside to inside. This voltage is caused by the cell membrane pumping potassium into the cell and sodium out of the cell. Despite the voltage drop being only 1 tenth of a volt, the electric field (voltage drop per metre) across the membrane is very high because the cell membrane is so thin. The electric field is, in fact, 10 million volts per meter (a very strong electric field).

Due to this very high electric field, the electrically charged molecules in the cell wall align themselves so that they are in a state of minimum energy. When the molecules are hit by a sound wave from outside, the molecule moves out of alignment of minimum energy. By an effect similar to the piezo-electric effect, the sound energy is converted into electro-magnetic energy of the same frequency. This process may occur from sound to electro-magnetic radiation or vice versa. The sound/ EM conversion is particularly important at ELF frequencies (1–300 Hz).

WHAT ARE THE COMMON ELECTROMAGNETIC HAZARDS?

Static electricity

Static electricity has a zero frequency and is caused by the build up of an electric charge on a non-conducting surface, for example the effect of friction on a rubber balloon. The electricity does not travel anywhere (hence, *static* electricity). Since static electricity often rises to thousands of volts, it gives rise to quite a strong electric field, hence the reason a rubber balloon will stick to a wall.

Static electricity is produced by TV and VDU screens, nylon carpets and clothes, plastics and air conditioning systems. These materials frequently occur in modern air conditioned offices. Static electricity is a common problem in these buildings and no doubt contributes to the Sick Building Syndrome. This condition is discussed in greater depth on page 185.

Static electricity may be greatly reduced by avoiding:

- Modern air conditioned buildings furnished with synthetic carpets, plastics;
- Rooms full of TV sets and VDUs;
- Wearing clothes made from nylon and other synthetic fibres. Natural fibres help to reduce your personal load of static electricity.

However, most people are unable to change their office and its furnishings and the more practical solution is to use an ionizer. Air in cities and office blocks usually has an excess of positive ions. An ionizer creates negative ions and restores the balance giving a slight excess of negative ions.

Weather systems sometimes produce an excess of positive charges in winds e.g. the Chinook in western Canada, the Sharav in Israel, the Foehn in Switzerland, Southern Germany and Austria, the Mistral in France, and the Sirocco in Italy. Ill health is more common in these regions during the time that these winds blow.

The ionizer causes dust to settle, mood to improve and many other allergic conditions, for example hayfever, asthma and catarrh, and migraine to get better. An ionizer does not help everyone, but it is particularly useful for the 30 per cent of the population who are 'weather sensitive' i.e. worse before thunderstorms. Modern ionizers no longer produce ozone as earlier models did. Ionizers cannot be promoted for health purposes in the United States, due to their benefits being overexaggerated in the past.

Direct Current

Direct current also has zero frequency. Direct current is used in many industrial processes such as electroplating, electrolysis, DC motors and electric furnaces. The last application often uses very high currents with a consequently very high magnetic field, which is a worrying health hazard for people working close by.

ELF (Extra Low Frequencies 1–300 Hz)

Naturally occurring ELF frequencies, e.g. Schumann waves, are relatively weak. By far the commonest source of ELF frequencies in the western world is mains electricity, and the numerous household devices that use it.

Mains frequency electricity flowing in wires creates electric and magnetic fields at the same frequency. The magnetic fields are more damaging to health than the electric fields. The magnetic field is related to the current

used by the device, but also whether or not the device creates a magnetic field for its operation as, for example, do motors and transformers. The higher the current and the more current used in windings, the higher the magnetic field. Household items that need the highest current are heating devices, followed by motorized devices, followed by lighting devices. The fields are particularly high very close to the device (within 6 inches). The background level, more than 6 feet away from most domestic devices, is very low.

The magnetic and electric field may be increased due to an effect called *perturbation* (magnification or diminution of the field). Perturbation usually increases the electric field around curved objects, e.g. the skull. Perturbation of the magnetic field also occurs due to metallic, especially iron-containing objects. A perturbed field can be up to a hundred times stronger than an unperturbed field.

Common sources of high electric and magnetic fields are:

Electric hair dryers

This device consists of both a motor and a heater with a consequently high magnetic field. In a hair dryer the magnetic and electric fields are applied directly to the brain, which is the most electrically sensitive organ in the body. Metal hair clips worn in the hair further perturb the field.

Motors

All devices containing motors, from electric clocks to fans, have a strong magnetic field surrounding them because of current passing through windings to induce a magnetic field to make the device work.

Shavers

The magnetic and electric fields in a shaver are solely due to the motor. This is held in close contact to the face with a high resultant field passing through the brain.

Electric overblankets

This is a heating device kept on all night. Although the current is not particularly high the wire is very close to the body and the electric blanket has a large surface area covering the whole body. It is also left on all night. The overall dose is, consequently, very high and these devices commonly cause cramp and increase the risk of miscarriages. They also cause problems because the hot plastic coated wires release chemical fumes, which are themselves toxic.

Heated water beds

These have a similar risk to electric overblankets.

High voltage power lines

Many people live under or close to high voltage power lines (60,000 people in United Kingdom). They are consequently exposed to electric and magnetic fields all the time that they are at home. It is strongly advisable to have *at least* the following separations between your house and high voltage power lines:

Voltage carried by line	Minimum advised separation
50,000 volts	200 feet
132,000 volts	300 feet
275,000 volts	500 feet
400,000 volts	750 feet

The electric field immediately under a high voltage power line can be strong enough to light an ordinary fluorescent tube held vertically at ground level, unconnected to the power line. (This experiment is potentially very dangerous and must not be attempted by people who are not experienced electrical engineers, because it is possible for currents to pass from the high voltage power line to earth with fatal results.)

The electric field from the high voltage power lines can be completely removed by covering the cable with an earthed screen. Burying the cable also reduces the magnetic field because the three cables are placed very close together and cancel out each other's field. The only safe way to reduce magnetic fields to very low levels is to move away from the cable. A moratorium on buildings under or near high voltage power lines is long overdue. In areas where housing has already been built, high voltage power lines should be put under ground and/or re-routed.

Transformers

These occur at the beginning and end of transmission lines. They step-up the generated voltage to transmission line voltage and step-down the voltage to the 240 volts domestic supply level. They are the source of strong magnetic fields and should be sited away from housing and work areas.

Motors and generators

These cause a very high magnetic field and may have a dangerous effect on people working in close proximity, e.g. electric motor mechanics, drivers of electric vehicles, power station workers and electric supply and maintenance engineers.

Ultra low frequency

The Navy has a technical problem in communicating with its submarines while they are under water. Ordinary radio waves will not pass through water. However, extra low frequency and ultra low frequency will pass through sea water. It is believed that ELF and ULF Navy transmitters may cause illnesses such as cot deaths. There is, not surprisingly, great secrecy about the location, power and frequency of these transmitters. As a general rule, however, for many reasons it is unwise to live close (within 10 miles), to any sort of military installation.

Radio, TV, CBs, radar, microwave transmitters and mobile phones (radio and microwaves)

Radio, TV, CB and microwave transmitters, and mobile phones all emit electrical and magnetic fields. The wavelength used is much shorter than ELF and when the frequency is above 30 GHz (10^9 Hz) the electrical and magnetic fields are measured, not in volts per centimetre and tesla, but in watts per square centimetre. The present official 'safe' level (10 milliwatts per square centimetre) is probably 1,000 times higher than the real 'safe' level (10 micro watts per square centimetre).

Consequently, there are many people working with, or living close to, these transmitters who are at an increased risk of sustaining cataracts, cancer, leukaemia, infertility and allergies, and conceiving children with Down's Syndrome. The risk of a transmitter causing problems is dependent on:

- the power of the transmitter in watts;
- the distance from the transmitter and the direction in which it is broadcasting. Being in the direct 'line of sight' of a transmitter that is broadcasting, greatly increases the risk (e.g. living at the end of a runway in the beam of a radar);
- the time exposed to the transmitter (in hours per day and number of years).

Microwave ovens (decimetre wavelength)

These ovens use the heating (thermal) effect of microwaves. The oven is a moderately powerful microwave transmitter, operating a frequency of 2.45 GHz. It beams EM waves at the food to be cooked. This frequency causes water molecules in the food to flip back and forth billions of times a second and this causes heating.

The microwave heating occurs simultaneously all through the item in the beam and microwave ovens, unlike ordinary ovens, heat from the inside outwards. Dangerous levels of microwaves are not detected when they are heating your body from the inside because heat is detected only by superficial nerves in the skin. Deep tissues have no heat sensing nerves. The microwave damage is worst in the parts of the body that have no blood supply to cool them, e.g. lenses in the eye.

Microwave ovens are unsatisfactory for two reasons:

- Sometimes they leak microwaves (this may be caused by damage to the door).
- They have very short cooking times and do not adequately kill germs. The rise in food poisoning cases over the past decade can be partly attributed to failure of microwave ovens adequately to sterilize food.

Visual Display Units (VDUs)

These emit static electricity, radiowaves, microwaves, infra-red, light, ultra-violet and x-rays. They are known to cause headaches, eye strain and skin problems. In women they have also been shown to increase the risk of miscarriage and they probably increase malformations. It is not known exactly how VDUs cause problems. It may be due to the magnetic field produced by the horizontal and vertical deflection coils in the cathode ray tube. The electric field can be reduced considerably by Gaussian screening, consisting of a cover of copper or aluminium foil around the outside of the VDU, grounded to earth.

Other ways of reducing the risk of VDUs include:

- Sensible positioning of VDUs, so that the operator is not close to lots of other machines. The magnetic and electric fields from the side and the back of VDUs are often worse than the fields from the front;
- Switching the machine off when not in use;
- Not using the VDU for more than 4 hours a day;
- Not using the VDU for more than one hour in continual use without a 15 minute break;
- Not working on a VDU during pregnancy. Ideally don't work on the VDU for 3 months *before* conception (this applies to both women and men).

Alternative low-radiation VDUs, including LCD and TFT screens, are now available but have not been widely adopted. It is to be hoped that the VDU work practices of Australia will soon be more widely adopted. These allow pregnant women to change to non-VDU work without any loss of pay, seniority or promotion prospects.

Fluorescent Lighting

Ordinary fluorescent lights, unlike sunlight, do not produce the full spectrum of visible light (i.e. from infra-red to ultra-violet). Some people working in buildings without windows are made ill by the narrow spectrum fluorescent light. Health returns if full spectrum fluorescent tubes or incandescent bulbs are used. Full spectrum light is also useful to treat a condition called 'Seasonal Affective Disorder', which occurs in some people during months with short hours of sunlight, in particular in higher latitudes, for example, parts of Scandinavia.

Sun bathing and sunbeds (ultra-violet light)

Every day the earth is being bombarded by ultra-violet light from the sun. Fortunately, only about 1 per cent of this ultra-violet energy gets through to the surface of the earth. The rest is filtered out by the ozone layer, which is located between 12 and 30 miles above the earth's surface.

Ultra-violet light has a wavelength of less than 4×10^{-7}m and, consequently, is an ionizing radiation. It is able to cause a particularly nasty form of cancer called melanoma, and also cataracts.

Ultra-violet light can be divided into three forms:

Ultra-violet A (wavelength 400 to 320 nm)
Ultra-violet B (wavelength 320 to 280 nm)
Ultra-violet C (wavelength 280 to 200 nm)

Most of the ultra-violet light in sunlight is UVA. UVB is up to 100 times more dangerous than UVA. Sunbeds usually radiate UVA but many may give out five times as much as would be expected from bright sunlight at the equator. Sunbeds should not be used, since they increase the risk of skin cancer by about nine times, especially in fair-skinned people.

You will receive increased levels of ultra-violet radiation in the following places:

- Near the equator where the sun's rays are close to vertical, and consequently stronger;
- On mountains where there is less cloud and atmosphere to absorb UV light;
- At the poles, where there has been destruction of the ozone layer due to CFCs from aerosols;
- In snowy locations and on beaches where ultra-violet light is reflected back from the ground.

Your risk of sustaining a melanoma is dependent on your skin type and your degree of exposure to UV light.

Your skin type

The darker your natural skin colour and the more easily you tan, the greater your resistance to melanomas. As a general rule, the closer a race (usually) lives to the equator, the darker their skin.

Your exposure to UV light

You have control over this factor by avoiding sunbathing and other UV hazards. A problem occurs when light-skinned people from temperate zones go to live in hot countries with little cloud cover, e.g. South Africa, Australia.

The commonest skin cancer produced by UV light is called a melanoma. The signs of a melanoma include:

An increase in size of an existing mole or appearance of a new one;
An irregular border to the mole;
Variation in colour across a mole;
Itching or bleeding from a mole;
A mole bigger than 5mm across.

If you have any of the above symptoms or signs, *please see your doctor immediately.*

Medical X-rays

X-rays increase the risk of cancer and other diseases. *There is no safe dose.* Risk is cumulative and depends on lifetime exposure, general state of health, and total load of neotoxins.

It is wise to follow these rules:

● Don't have any X-ray investigations that you can avoid. If you do have an X-ray, wear a lead shield over testes or ovaries;

● For women, don't have any X-ray investigation if you could possibly be pregnant (i.e. have the X-ray within 10 days of the start of your last period);

● For men *and* women, don't have any X-ray investigations unless absolutely essential for three months prior to conception of a child as both the sperm and the egg will be maturing during this time.

● Try to avoid X-raying infants and young

children since a single X-ray has more chance of causing a cancer over the following 70 years.

Nuclear reactors, reprocessing plants and military installations (X-rays and gamma rays)

There is no 'safe' level of radiation. Radiation exposure is cumulative over your lifetime, and the greater the dose the greater the risk of illness. The X-ray and gamma ray radiation sources are:

Cosmic rays from space that pass through the ionosphere;
Gamma rays from building materials (e.g. plaster);
Radon gas (see next section);
Medical exposure (from X-rays, body scans and radio isotopes);
Occupational (X-rays and radio isotopes);
Domestic exposure (e.g. luminous dials and smoke detectors);
Fall out from nuclear weapons;
Discharges from nuclear reactors and reprocessing plants.

In areas close to nuclear reactors, reprocessing plants, in spite of reassurance to the contrary, the incidence of childhood leukaemias is between 5 and 10 times greater than the national average. Adult illness in these areas is less likely to show such a marked variation from the national average, because there is a latency of at least 5 to 15 years between exposure to radiation and seeing its full effect.

Another problem is that the long-term side-effects of radiation have been grossly underestimated. Radiation workers are 2 to 3 times more likely to develop cancer than was previously estimated.

The soil and beaches near reactors and reprocessing plants are subject to accidental spillage, and deliberate discharges of nuclear materials. The Irish Sea around Sellafield is the most radioactive in the world. It is unwise to live within 30 miles of a nuclear reactor or reprocessing plant, or to eat seafood caught in such areas. This advice is of particular importance to children and people of child-bearing age.

Radon

Radon[222] is a heavy, colourless, odourless gas released from granite and similar rocks. It decays to rapidly to form polonium[210], which emits alpha radiation. Although alpha waves do not penetrate tissue very deeply, polonium is breathed into the lungs, where it is likely to cause lung cancer, especially in smokers.

Radon enters the basements of houses from surrounding soil and water, building materials, cracks in the foundations and other breaks in foundations where pipes enter. The official danger level for radon in the United Kingdom has recently been reduced to 200 becquerels per cubic foot of air, although this is probably still too high.

Radon gas accumulation can be prevented by:

- Stopping radon gas entering the house by raising the pressure in the basement with a fan. This then forces radon *out* of the house;
- Sealing basement cracks around foundations and pipes;
- Providing separate ventilation to the basement. The air from the basement should not communicate with the rest of the house;
- The drains that pass through the basement should vent to the outside;
- Try not to live in a radon area, but if you do, don't have defective foundations;
- Be careful of deep wells, which may provide a path for the gas to come to the surface from radon-bearing rocks many feet beneath the earth.

Cosmic Radiation (UV rays, X-rays and gamma rays)

The earth is constantly bombarded with cosmic radiation from outer space. You are protected from the full effect of this radiation by the ozone layer which absorbs a large proportion of this radiation. The protective effect of the atmosphere is reduced at the north and south poles, due to the destructive effect of CFCs on the ozone layer.

At high altitude, aircrews and frequent air travellers sustain an increased dose of cosmic radiation. Airliners cruise at 30,000 feet (6 miles high) and at this altitude, the level of dangerous rays is far higher than at sea level. The levels of cosmic radiation are also increased at times of maximum sunspot activity, which occur every 11 years (1979, 1990, 2001).

SOUND

Sound and vibration are detected by the ear, but may have an effect on the whole body. If you are exposed to high noise levels you are more likely to suffer from many illnesses, including allergies, angina and heart attacks. Sound and electromagnetic waves are interchangeable, and sounds of frequency of 1 to 30 Hz are converted to electromagnetic waves at the cell membranes. These ELF frequencies damage the body, since it also uses these low frequencies for brainwaves and nerve transmission.

Occupational deafness is a high risk for military personnel, shipbuilders, quarriers, pneumatic drillers, bottlers, weavers, wood-workers, printers and many factory workers. In almost every case, damage to the ears can be avoided by using quieter but more expensive processes. However, the pain and suffering caused to workers, and their health bills, don't enter into the calculation of production costs. Consequently, there is no incentive to make these jobs less noisy and more safe. If you do work in a noisy job, always wear ear protectors.

Does ultrasound scanning cause health problems?

Ultrasound scans are now used routinely in pregnancy. When used at 16 weeks they can measure the size of the baby's head and confirm the age of pregnancy in weeks.

It is possible that ultrasound scans may be dangerous for two reasons:

1. They are used during the first 12 weeks of pregnancy when all the major systems of the baby are being formed. At this time tissues are particularly susceptible to malformations. The energy produced by an ultrasound scanner is sufficient to cause bubble formation (cavitation) in a test tube of water. There is no guarantee that cavitation does not permanently damage developing tissues.
2. The beam of ultrasound is directed at the skull about half an inch in front of the ears. A high frequency (1 MHz) ultrasound scan may damage the developing ears, which are the part of the body most sensitive to sound. The deteriorating level of hearing in young people has been blamed on excessive exposure to rock music. This may be partly true, but since the majority of today's teenagers were scanned in their mothers' wombs, the damage to hearing may have been started by ultrasound.

GEOPATHIC STRESS

Geopathic stress is probably caused by extra low frequency (ELF) earth rays coming from the ground, and may make you ill. You are most vulnerable to these rays in bed, because you remain relatively still for 8 hours, and have less resistance when you are asleep. Geopathic stress is able to produce most of the classical allergic symptoms, including:

- Persistent tiredness which is not relieved by rest or sleep. The sufferer wakes up in the morning exhausted or depressed;
- Poor weight gain due to reduced appetite and even nausea in the morning;
- Palpitations or rapid pulse and also muscle cramps;
- Excessive sweating.

Other symptoms and diseases, many of which are related to sleep, include:

- Insomnia and disturbed sleep, e.g. nightmares;
- Finding reasons for not going to bed or getting out of bed, e.g. sleep walking;
- Feeling very cold in bed and shivery;
- Children are particularly sensitive to geopathic stress. They will sleep in a very uncomfortable position if it means they can move away from earth rays. They also may refuse to sleep in their own bed and move to the safer bed of a brother or sister, or parent.

Geopathic stress can stop the immune and detoxification systems from working properly. Long-term exposure to earth rays can cause cancer. German studies have shown a very strong connection between cancer and the part of the body exposed to earth rays.

Geopathic rays are caused by underground streams. Occasionally the underground streams will cross, and the point above the crossing will be particularly dangerous.

If you think that you or your children may be affected by geopathic stress, then try moving the bed or cot to a completely different position or room. If geopathic stress is the cause you should see an improvement in a week.

How can I tell the position of underground streams and earth rays?

The best way to find the position of underground streams and earth rays is to get an experienced dowser to find them for you. Dowsers are people who are able to find these streams by learning to become very sensitive to tiny changes in magnetic fields. If you don't have the services of a dowser, then animals and plants may be able to help you.

Some animals and plants dislike earth rays and will move or grow away from them (earth ray avoiders); other animals and plants are the opposite and actually seek out earth rays (earth ray seekers). Animals are far more useful in detecting these rays as they will move away, or towards, the earth rays, according to their preference. If earth ray avoider animals are made to stay over earth rays, especially crossing points, they will become ill and may even die. Plants cannot move away from earth rays, so they either fail to germinate or grow irregularly, or lopsidedly, or without fruit, or lose their bark or develop strange lumps.

Table 4.3 gives the earth ray avoiders and earth ray seekers.

If you suspect that a point in your house, for example your bed, is subject to earth rays, carry out this simple test. Put a dog on your bed or easychair. If the dog will not stay in that position, or if an 'earth ray avoider' houseplant (azalea, begonia, cactus) withers when placed there, then resite the bed or easychair. Retry the test to confirm a new safe position.

This phenomenon of earth rays was very

Table 4.3		Earth ray avoiders	Earth ray seekers
Animals		Dog	Cat
		Cows	Bees
		Horses	Ants
		Pigs	Bacteria
		Chickens	Fungi
		Birds (nesting)	Parasites
Trees		Apple	Cherry
		Pear	Plum
		Beech	Peach
		Nut	Elderberry
		Lilac	Mistletoe
Plants		Currant bushes	Asparagus
		Sunflower	
		Houseplants	
		Azaleas	
		Begonias	
		Cacti	

well known to our ancestors, who took great care to site important buildings, e.g. churches and big houses, on sites that had no adverse earth rays.

SUMMARY

- Electricity may cause allergic symptoms due to the effect of electric and magnetic fields. Electrical sensitivity is much commoner in people who already have food allergies and/or chemical sensitivities.

- All electromagnetic radiations are part of a very, very broad spectrum; they have largely similar properties and differ only in their wavelength. The wavelength and frequency are related by the formula:

$$\text{wavelength} = \frac{\text{speed of light}}{\text{frequency}}$$

- Electromagnetic radiation with a wavelength of greater than 4×10^{-7}m is termed non-ionizing radiation (NIR). Electromagnetic radiation with a wavelength of less than 4×10^{-7}m is termed ionizing radiation (IR) and can produce ionization in molecules that it hits. The effect of NIR and IR is additive, and the greater the total dose of radiation, the greater the risk of illness or allergy.

- Dose of EM radiation =

$$\begin{array}{ccc} \text{strength of} & \times & \text{`proximity' to} & \times & \text{time} \\ \text{source} & & \text{source of} & & \text{exposed} \\ \text{(amount of} & & \text{neotoxin} & & \text{to} \\ \text{neotoxin} & & & & \text{neotoxin} \\ \text{at source)} & & & & \end{array}$$

- An electric field is created by an electric voltage, and a magnetic field is created by an electric current. Electric fields can be screened by a Gaussian screen, whereas magnetic fields are very difficult to screen.

- The likelihood of suffering from electrical sensitivity is dependent on the frequency, coherence and waveform of the EM wave striking the body. The intensity of a wave is less important, provided that it is greater than the threshold level.

- Electrically sensitive people give out radiation, and electrical equipment may fail to operate properly for them.

- Sound waves can be converted to EM waves at the cell membrane due to a phenomenon resembling the piezo-electric effect.

- Geopathic stress caused by earth rays can cause allergic illness.

- To reduce your total load of physical neotoxins, apply as many of the following suggestions as you can:
  1. Try not to live or work near a high voltage power line, electric motor, generator or transformer, transmitter, nuclear reactor or reprocessing plant, or military installations.
  2. Reduce your exposure to electric and magnetic fields by turning off all devices when not in use, for example turn of VDUs and don't use them for more than 4 hours a day, or more than an hour at a time without a break.
  3. Particularly avoid using electric over-blankets, heater water beds, micro-wave ovens and sunbeds.

4. Don't have any unnecessary X-ray investigations, especially in the 3 months before conception.
5. Reduce your work and home sound level so that you can easily have a conversation in a normal speaking voice.
6. Review your sleeping place to see if it may be subject to geopathic stress.
7. Reduce your total load of neotoxins.
8. Particularly remove the neotoxin(s) to which you are most susceptible.
9. Use sleep and rest, exercise, vitamins, minerals and other supplements to help yourself back to complete health.

CHAPTER FIVE

MENTAL NEOTOXINS: STRESS AND YOUR HEALTH

One of the most underrated factors causing suffering and exacerbation of allergies is mental stress. If you take ten typical consultations with a family doctor, the real reason that at least half the patients come to see him or her is because they are overstressed and unhappy with their life. Although these patients may have allergies or other physical symptoms, often these symptoms are relatively minor, and the illnesses will last only two or three days. It is the patient's stress level that decides whether a patient consults the doctor or just soldiers on.

There is a sound biochemical explanation to explain the effect of stress and mood. When you are happy your body produces more of the substances called endorphins, which are natural pain-killers and anti-depressants. The happier you are, the higher your endorphin level and the higher your threshold to pain and distress. Conversely, when you are stressed, unhappy and have negative thoughts, these can generate the same free radicals which cause cell damage and allergic problems.

WHAT IS STRESS?

Stress is the original term used by Professor Hans Selye when he described his General Adaption Syndrome (GAS) mentioned on page 33. Stress is the body's reaction to a damaging outside factor (a neotoxin), which causes an internal effect. Stress is a mental neotoxin, and on its own can produce the classical allergy symptoms which include persistent tiredness, swelling, palpitations and sweating.

Stress may also precipitate or exacerbate existing allergic conditions, such as asthmas, colitis and migraine.

What are the sources of stress?

In less civilized times, the causes of stress would have been:

Starvation and hunger
The effects of weather
Pain
Haemorrhage
Wild animals
Civil and military disturbances

In present times, apart from the increasing number of people falling through the social security net, these problems have been replaced with:

● Stress from emotional problems (unhappiness, loneliness, bereavement);
● Stress at work (repeated deadlines, interruptions, threat of redundancy);
● Stress at home (domestic problems financial pressures);

- Stress during leisure (social pressure to keep up with fashion);
- General stress (crime, invasion of privacy etc.).

Although few of these are directly life-threatening, the amount of reserve, i.e., the amount of energy, patience and health left to deal with an unexpected crisis has been reduced. The sources of stress and reduction in reserve are represented in Figure 5.1, early and late twentieth century stress circles. The couple in the late twentieth century stress circle are good candidates for allergies and illness, through being under such great stress. Their reserve, which allows them to cope with further stress, is vanishingly small and there are very few resources left to deal with an unexpected crisis.

An analogy for the position of the man or the woman in the late-twentieth century stress circle is that of a person who is given the task of filling a bath, when he or she has control of the taps, but no control over the plughole.

How does stress affect the body?

Stress affects the body via the brain. The brain then activates two systems, the sympathetic autonomic system and the hypothalamus pituitary and adrenal cortex system.

The sympathetic autonomic system

The autonomic nervous system is responsible for all the unconscious body functions, e.g. breathing, heart rate and bowels. The sympathetic system is responsible for producing the high state of arousal (fight or flight). This arousal is caused by release of adrenalin from the adrenal medulla. The adrenalin initially has a stimulating affect on the immune and detoxification systems.

The hypothalamus, pituitary, and adrenal cortex system

The brain acts on the hypothalamus, which instructs the pituitary to release the hormone ACTH (Adrenocortotrophic Hormone). The ACTH travels in the blood to the adrenal cortex (outside of the adrenal), where it causes the release of the steroid cortisol. Cortisol initially has a stimulating effect on the immune system.

The effect of the adrenalin and cortisol is initially stimulatory (a valuable response in an emergency or infection). The problem arises when stimulation becomes prolonged and the body remains constantly aroused in a state of 'fight or flight'. If this over-stimulation continues, even while asleep, then the body starts to show allergic symptoms and to become more susceptible to the other neotoxins (biological, chemical and physical).

What happens to a body that is overstressed?

Figure 5.3 illustrates the different stages the body (or an organ) passes through when subjected to increasing levels of stress. Initially there is a phase of sub-optimal efficiency, when the body is not really stretched. If stress occurs this is followed by a phase of optimal efficiency, where the body is at its most efficient and all systems are working well but below full capacity.

If stress continues to rise, the body enters a phase of fatigue and exhaustion, and levels of efficiency drop. If stress level increases still further then the body reaches a point of collapse. The objective in life is to be operating in the phase of optimal efficiency so that the body is neither under nor over stressed.

Why is stress so poorly appreciated?

There are many reasons for stress being so poorly appreciated. These reasons include:

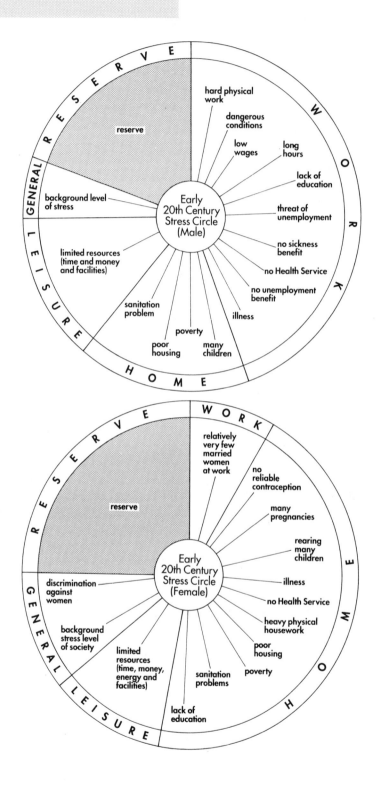

Figure 5.1

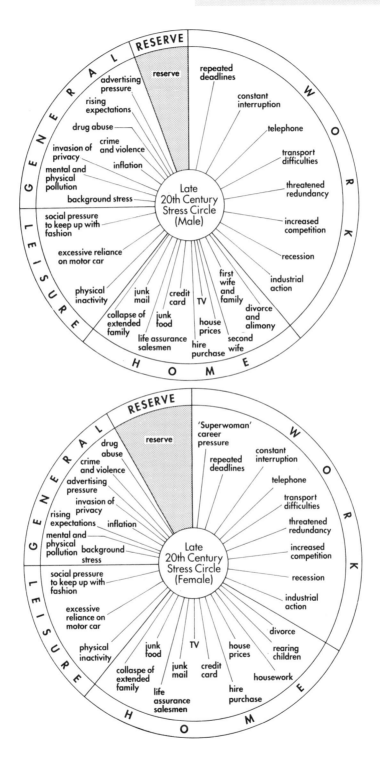

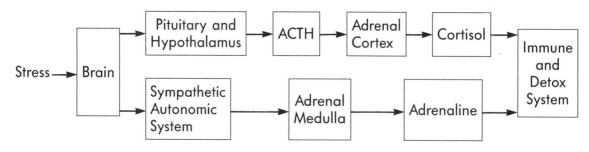

Figure 5.2 **How stress affects the body**

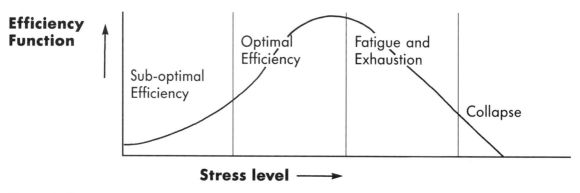

Figure 5.3

- The fact that stress generated in an individual is more dependent upon the person's response rather than the situation, e.g. a television appearance that might bring blind panic to one individual would be welcomed in a calm and relaxed manner by another. Thus the stress is not so much the *situation* itself but rather the *response* to that situation.
- The problem with stress is not merely the *quantity*, but also its *quality*: there is good stress (stimulation or fulfilment), and bad stress (anger or frustration). It appears that the latter is far more likely to cause stress and to act as a neotoxin. The former may actually promote good health.
- There is no objective measure of stress, as there is for the concentration of a poisonous

gas in the atmosphere or the intensity of an electromagnetic field. The usual arbiter of stress is a doctor – who is a member of a profession notorious for its high-stress working practices. Consequently, the condition is greatly underdiagnosed.

How is stress associated with allergy?

Before becoming ill, stress-prone people frequently suffer from frustration, depression, and demonstrate anxiety and nervousness when under pressure. They may also experience an abnormal and deepening fatigue, not refreshed by sleep, and achieve little despite working long hours (60 hours plus). They often have several jobs, but their work is surrounded with insecurity, feelings of inadequacy and inability to cope. It is common that in the three to six months before the start of an allergy there is an abrupt change in circumstances or life event (see long-term stress). The greater this change, the shorter the interval between the life event and the onset of the allergy.

Stress can be further classified into:

- *Short-term stress* – this is caused by hour-to-hour events and is fairly easy to appreciate. This type of stress can be best analysed by keeping a stress diary (see page 119). To reduce short-term stress, you must precisely define your objectives, and make the best use of your time and resources.
- *Long-term stress* – this is caused by life events. It is well recognized that obviously negative events cause stress, e.g. death of a close friend or spouse, divorce or separation, going to jail, trouble with the police, accident or injury, financial or legal problems, employment or redundancy. However, apparently positive events are also stressful, e.g. marriage, job promotion and rise in salary, moving to a new house, family readjustment, pregnancy, retirement, changing schools, and holidays.

As a general rule, the more changes that you have in any year, the more stressed you are and more likely to suffer an allergy or illness. With short-term or long-term stress, it is often a relatively minor event that causes the final collapse (the straw that breaks the camel's back), and causes the onset of an allergy.

Do isolated rural communities in the Third World suffer from stress?

Stress is especially a western disease. It occurs because of the high pace of life and competitiveness for recognition, from the cradle to the grave. Allergies are unknown in Brazilian rainforest communities, where the social structure, religious beliefs and the extended family act as a far better support system than we have in the 'civilized' world.

For many people in the western world, there is an increasing gap between their real personality and the person that they are expected to be. Eventually, some individuals find it too difficult to sustain the image of the person that they are supposed to be, and lapse into an illness which is often an allergy.

What are the sources of stress in Western society?

The important point to remember is that the stress arises not so much from the situation, as from your response to that situation.

Common stress provoking situations at work

Overwork (especially over 50 hours a week); more than one job; financial problems; too much or too little responsibility; problems with colleagues, subordinates and bosses; too much pressure and repeated deadlines; periods of unemployment or threatened redundancy; lack of recognition or support; frustrating work practices; night shifts; relocation and travel problems; legal problems.

Common stress problems at home

Relationship problems; family disagreement; housing problems; high population density; illness and death of relatives; looking after children and relatives; financial problems; legal problems.

Why do so many people in middle management suffer from stress?

The middle manager's place in the management pyramid is the reason for his, or her, stress. There are directors issuing unreasonable directives from above, and the shop floor making unreasonable demands for the available resources from below. The middle management's job is often to try to to reconcile the irreconcilable, usually at the expense of his or her own health.

Why do high-flying executives suffer from stress?

'Yuppies' suffer from stress because their working practices and working conditions are not conducive to good health. They are often working in air conditioned, sealed buildings full of fixtures giving out formaldehyde. This gives them a large load of chemical neotoxins. They often use mobile phones that irradiate their brains, and their work practices epitomize stress, with constant minute-by-minute deadlines and enormous interpersonal competition. They often have to commute long distances and work long hours. This lifestyle is an ideal formula for stress, and this makes them particularly vulnerable to allergies, including ME – often called 'yuppie flu'. Yuppies pay a high health price because of the method of earning their money.

Why do shop floor workers in unskilled jobs suffer from stress?

Boring, monotonous jobs are often very stressful because there is little fulfilment from completing each task. This is especially the case if there is shift work and if the environment is very hot, very cold, or wet, since in all these cases the body has to work much harder to cope. Despite these negative factors, these jobs are also less well paid, thus often causing financial anxieties.

Is having less money stressful?

Every single survey has shown that people with less money die younger and suffer more illness during their shorter life. This problem is not only related to having less money, but also less education and a higher consumption of alcohol, tobacco and fast food. You can make best use of your money by giving up smoking, drinking only moderate amounts of alcohol and trying to eat fresh organic foods rather than convenience foods.

Which personality is more likely to suffer from stress and allergies?

It has been found that illness and some allergies are more common amongst a certain type of personality, arbitrarily labelled Type A.

Type A personality

Type A Personality is the fist clenching, desk banging executive type, constantly fighting to achieve more and more in less and less time. These personalities (usually men) have a very high drive, often towards poorly defined goals, with consequent 'free floating anxiety'. They have 'hurry sickness' and a great eagerness to compete and be recognized. They will refuse to acknowledge tiredness or fatigue, thus taking them past the point at which they start to become liable to serious disease.

Characteristically, type A personalities are very impatient, refuse to queue and walk, talk and eat at the double. Type A personalities tend to live life in the fast lane, and smoke, drink, and eat too much. On average they have a higher blood pressure which in the early stages can usually be brought back to normal by reducing the total load of neotoxins.

Type B personality

Type B personalities are far more relaxed and have a far more philosophical response to potential stressful situations. They are more aware of their body's fatigue and rest when tired. They are rewarded for their temperate personalities by being less likely to suffer from allergies and illness.

How can I tell if I am overstressed?

For short-term events it is best assessed by keeping a stress diary as shown in Table 5.1.

For long-term events, you will need to look at the number of major and minor changes that have occurred in your life in the past year. The greater the number of changes, domestic, work, social, financial, interpersonal, occurring in a 12-month period, the greater

---

Table 5.1 **Stress diary**

Day: .... Date: ....

Time	Activity	Stress level (Rate 1–4)	Quality of Stress (+ or –)
0–7am			
7am			
8am			
9am			
10am			
11am			
Noon			
1pm			
2pm			
3pm			
4pm			
5pm			
6pm			
7pm			
8pm			
9pm			
10pm			
11pm			
m'night			

Rate your stress level 1–4

Stress level
1 = slight stress
2 = moderate stress
3 = great stress
4 = very great stress

Quality of stress + = (stimulation or fulfilment)
− = (anger or frustration)

the likelihood of serious disease (see list in *the superhealth plan* page 132).

What symptoms are caused by stress?

- A frequent feeling of frustration or anger;
- Inability to concentrate or make simple decisions;
- Inability to relax or to switch off;
- Inability to cope or finish jobs;
- Irrational behaviour;
- A feeling of anxiety and/or depression and loss of self confidence;
- Irrational fear or even outright panic;
- An increase or reduction in appetite;
- Loss of sex drive;
- Difficulty in getting to sleep or early morning wakening;
- Weakness, tiredness or lethargy;
- Fear of disease or death.

What changes in behaviour are caused by stress?

- Increase in smoking;
- Increased intake of prescribed or over-the-counter drugs;
- Increase in alcohol intake;
- Uncharacteristic aggression or type A behaviour;
- Excess hand or teeth clenching;
- Explosive mannerisms;
- Reckless driving;
- Increased or decreased appetite;
- Increased or decreased sleep;
- Memory or concentration impairment.

WHAT CAN I DO TO HANDLE STRESS BETTER?

In order to handle stress, you must fully understand what stress is (see above for descriptions of symptoms and behavioural effects of stress). Many people are unwittingly walking around with ideal recipes for stress inside their heads, because they are constantly working towards poorly defined objectives. They consequently have no means of telling if and when they have achieved the vague task that they have set themselves. For example 'I want to be successful' – what does successful mean? A large house (how large?) A big car (is a Rolls Royce big enough?), an exotic holiday (is the Bahamas OK?).

They may also have totally unreasonable expectations:

$$\text{Stress} = \frac{\text{expectations}}{\text{achievements}}$$

Stress occurs when the expectations are far greater than the achievements.

In order to escape stress, and especially bad stress (anger and frustration), you must:

- Analyse your present life, and identify short-term and long-term stress and decide on optimum stress levels;
- Remove sources of stress;
- Change your response to stress, i.e. – don't just become cross, do something constructive, like changing your job, social situation, leisure habits and outlook.
- Use relaxation techniques to cope with stress.

If you are unhappy, deal with it in three stages:

1. The first step is the most important: this is to accept that you are unhappy, and to decide that you are going to do something positive to change it.
2. You need to set yourself a target of the one thing that you really want to do this year in order to make yourself happy. Write down exactly what it is you want to do and put the details in a scrapbook together with pictures, so that you can visualize it very accurately. If you've decided that your

problem is that you're overweight, then write down a description of exactly the weight you want to be and what you'll look like. Then cut out pictures of attractive slim people and stick the pictures and details into your scrapbook. Look at the book every day to reinforce what you're going to do. Remember if you don't have a dream then it's never going to come true.

3. Get rid of the mental blocks and the worries that are holding you back. Worrying has its place, but when it gets out of proportion then it stops you from progressing. The way that you control worry is simpler than you think. Write down exactly what your worries are. Be very specific. When you focus on the real problem you will find that there is actually very little holding you back. You'll also find that it's not so difficult to overcome the problems. When you've written down your exact worries then throw away the piece of paper and you'd be surprised how often the problem goes away.

Make sure that you have enough love and laughter in your life. If you don't have enough, then change the way that you live your life so that every day you laugh, and every day you smile at at least three people. Most people's impression of you is based on their first meeting with you and if you start off smiling your life becomes much easier. Few people have it within their power to be brilliant but almost everybody can be happy and pleasant.

How do I remove sources of stress?

● Decide on your very few *real objectives*. This is not easy, since most people are conditioned to work on the problem in front of them, rather than defining the real

problem, and then solving that. For example, my problem is not, 'How can I get these ten things done in the next hour', but, 'What things *need* to be done?' *Then* arrange to do just those two things. Many problems are merely in your own, and other people's, head.

● Prioritize activities and do important things first.

● Plan realistically and set sensible deadlines for the available resources of time, energy and money.

● Completely concentrate on, and enjoy doing, just one thing at a time.

● Ensure that your life is balanced. Having enough time for family and friends, exercise, hobbies and free unfilled time is important.

● Don't try to do everything yourself. Get the support of others at home and work. Discuss problems and communicate difficulties. Set realistic time limits and review progress regularly. Then let the other person get on with it, and don't be over critical.

● Know your own limitations, don't try to be superman or superwoman.

● Learn from your mistakes (and hopefully, the mistakes of others before they become your own).

● Give yourself regular holidays, adequate breaks at meal times, and sufficient sleep.

● Anticipate and avoid stressful situations.

How can I change my response to stress?

● Learn to assert yourself, while still remaining sensitive and sympathetic. Don't become angry and aggressive, but instead confidently but coolly insist on having your point of view considered.

● Don't overreact to small grievances, or continue to grumble about old sources of annoyance. Forget the past and don't bear grudges.

- Analyse your behaviour, and don't become stressed when you feel uncomfortable, awkward, frustrated or dependent. Instead, think positive and try to minimize your negative feelings.
- Accept life as it is, warts and all.

How can I cope with stress?

The following techniques will help you to cope with stress.

Exercise

Exercise reduces the circulating level of adrenalin and cortisol. It also promotes sweating and increases the circulation of blood through the liver and kidneys. Both of these clear biological, chemical, physical and mental neotoxins. It also promotes sleep and a relaxed state of mind.

Sleep

Lack of sleep is very stressful, as is working at a time when your body expects to be asleep (shift working). Sleep therapy, e.g. making sure that you have 10 hours rest in bed every night for a week is a greatly underused way to reduce stress. If you feel unwell for any reason, try giving yourself an extra 2 hours sleep a night until you feel better.

Natural relaxation

Use natural relaxation techniques (two twenty-minute sessions), and make them an integral part of your day, together with exercise and vitamins. See relaxation as part of your exercise programme. Try breathing exercises and consider taking up structured relaxation techniques like yoga, meditation, and self-hypnosis. All these techniques require 100 per cent commitment, and you can't do them with one eye on the clock, or when you are likely to be disturbed by the phone. Set aside a time and space that cannot be encroached upon by other activities or people. These relaxation techniques are then able to reverse the adverse effects of stress.

Sex

This can be very relaxing, but, as for meditation, requires enough time to be enjoyed and fully appreciated. However, sex does increase the load of allergic substances, especially for women, and this may adversely affect allergy sufferers, see page 29.

Relationships and love

A strong relationship with another person has been shown to be a very important factor in reducing the level and effects of stress. Having enough love in your life can help you cope with a lot of other physical problems. Being a member of an organization, group or church, is also beneficial in terms of stress management.

Finally, try to avoid 'instant' twentieth-century remedies to induce relaxation, such as tranquillizers, TV, cigarettes and alcohol. There *are* no short-cuts.

SUMMARY

- Stress can produce many allergic symptoms.
- The twentieth century is a potent source of stress for most people.
- Stress causes the release of adrenalin and cortisol from the adrenal gland. This first stimulates the immune and detoxification systems, but if stress persists for too long it may later cause a malfunction.

- Stress is caused not so much by the situation but the *response* to the situation. Stress may be 'good' stress (stimulation or fulfilment), or 'bad' stress (anger or frustration).
- Stress may be short-term or long-term. Short-term stress is caused by hour-to-hour events. Long-term stress is caused by life-events. Even apparently positive life-events are stressful. The more stress you have in one year, the more likely you are to be ill or suffer an allergy or sensitivity.
- Stress, on its own, may be responsible for allergic symptoms and changes in behaviour. To reduce stress you must make a change in your lifestyle to remove the sources of stress, and change your response to stress.
- Exercise, sleep, natural relaxation and sex, strong relationships and plenty of love will help you cope with stress.

CHAPTER SIX

YOUR SUPERHEALTH PLAN

THE SUPERHEALTH PLAN

If, after reading the list on page 20, you feel that you are suffering from an allergy, then you can try the Superhealth Plan.

For young people, a good pointer that indicates whether or not you suffer from allergies, is to look at the thickness of your NHS notes held by your GP. If you are under 40 years old and your notes are one inch or thicker (the thick file syndrome), then there is a strong likelihood that you have an allergic disease(s).

If you follow the Superhealth Plan you will reduce your total load of neotoxins. If you suffer from an allergy this will almost certainly produce a dramatic improvement in your health. The plan works by reversing the errors in lifestyle which have made you ill. There are two reasons why you may become ill.

- **A genetic problem**
  This is inherited from your parents. You cannot change your parents or remove the genetic problem from your body, but you can greatly reduce its effect by removing the factors that emphasize its presence, e.g. most of the effects of coeliac disease may be removed by completely excluding wheat and wheat products from the diet.
- **An acquired problem**
  This has occurred because of some error in lifestyle. The body has an enormous ability to heal itself, provided that the underlying cause of illness is removed. Whatever the cause of your illness, allergic or otherwise, 'The Superhealth Plan' will give your body the best chance to cure itself.

There are two stages in the Superhealth Plan:

1. **Self Assessment**
   This involves reviewing your present lifestyle by filling in the following question-naires, then identifying the activities, places and times when you may be suffering from neotoxins. You will have to follow the relevant chapter to see how to reduce that neotoxin.
2. **Superhealth lifestyle change**
   Change your lifestyle so that you get rid of the acquired problem. You can do this by following the three rules:

   a) reduce your total load of neotoxins.
   b) reduce particularly the neotoxin to which you are especially sensitive.
   c) Use sleep, rest, exercise, vitamins, minerals and other supplements to help yourself back to complete health.

The way to find out which neotoxin affects you is to fill in the following questionnaires, including the environmental diary, and to see which activity, place, and time causes your

THE SUPERHEALTH
SELF-ASSESSMENT (GENERAL)

Table 6.1 **General Self-assessment**

Name: .... Address: ....

Date of birth: .... Age: .... Tel: ....

Your height................... Your weight .... Your maximum weight ever...................

Summary of allergic problems

Date when last completely well:

Details of allergic problems: (see page 20 *22* for list)

Started: Symptoms following:

Previous medical problems

Accidents:

Operations:

Hospital treatment:

Allergies (e.g. hayfever/penicillin)

Medication (prescribed and over the counter):

Please list serious and allergic diseases occurring in your family

(See page 20 for list)

Mother:

Father:

Sisters:

Brothers:

Habits:

Smoking: Cigarettes per day

Are you a passive smoker?   Yes/No

Drinking: Units per week

(1 unit = half a pint of beer, 1 glass of wine, 1 measure of spirit)

Bowel

Do your motions smell unpleasant?   Yes/No

Do you suffer from much wind?   Yes/No

Does any other part of your body produce an unusual/unpleasant smell? Yes/No

allergic symptoms to get better or worse. It is helpful to split the day into thirds when you are going through the questionnaire, and to think about your load of neotoxins separately at work, home and hobbies, and during sleep. Each takes approximately 8 hours of your day.

FOOD

The first factor to look at is your diet. If you have not kept a diet diary (see page 43), then write down a list of *everything* that you eat and

drink in a typical day. Be sure to include snacks, write down what you really eat, not what you feel you ought to eat (see table 6.2).

It is very useful to divide up foods according to food families, to see how often you eat each food or food family. Fill in the diet inventory to see which foods and food families you repeat most often. If you are unsure which food family something belongs to, refer to the food family list on page 233. If a food makes you ill or feel 'high', put 'I' or 'H' in the appropriate box.

Table 6.2 **Diet Diary**

	Food	Drink	Symptoms
Breakfast			
Midmorning			
Lunch			
Midafternoon			
Tea			
Dinner			

Please specify source of food, putting a letter after it:

F = frozen
T = tinned
B = bottled
P = packet
U = unprocessed (i.e. none of the above)

Table 6.3 **Food questionnaire**

Food	Never eaten	Eaten once a month	Eaten 1–3 times a wk	Eaten every day
Wheat				
Wheat products				
Other cereals				
Milk				
Cheese				
Milk products				
Beef (all forms)				
Pork (all forms)				
Lamb				
Chicken				
Eggs				
Fish				
Citrus fruits				
Apples and pears				
Grapes				
Plums and peaches				
Melon				
Nuts				
Banana				
Berries				
Tomatoes				
Potatoes				
Peas and beans				
Soya (all forms)				
Onions and leeks				
Lettuce				
Cabbage				
Cauliflower				
Carrot				
Yeast				
Chocolate				

Drinks	Never drunk	Drunk once a month	Drunk 1–3 times a wk	Drunk every day
Alcoholic				
Soft drinks				
Fruit juices				
Coffee				
Tea				
Herb teas				
Tap water				

Miscellaneous	Never eaten	Eaten once a month	Eaten 1–3 times a wk	Eaten every day
Sauces				
Gravies				
Chutneys				
Sweets				
Food Additives (E numbers)				

Also make a list of foods for which you crave.
(i.e. that give you a lift and you like to take at
least once a day), and foods that make you ill.

Table 6.4 **Other biological neotoxins questionnaire**

Biological Neotoxin	Never exposed	Exposed once a month	Exposed 1–3 times a wk	Exposed every day
Cats				
Dogs				
Birds				
Feathers				
Other pets				
Grass pollen				
Flowers				
Weeds				
Tree pollen				
Indoor plants				

Biological Neotoxin	Never exposed	Exposed once a month	Exposed 1–3 times a wk	Exposed every day
Fungi				
Damp				
House dust mite				

Table 6.5 **Your water supply**

What is the source of your water supply? ....
(List Water Board and, if known, reservoir)

Does your water supply come from an area
where there is much bracken growing? Yes/No

spraying of crops? Yes/No

Do you have lead pipes in your house? Yes/No

Do you notice a change in your health when
you drink or cook in a different water supply? Yes/No

CHEMICAL NEOTOXINS

Fill in Table 6.6 to assess how often you are exposed to chemical neotoxins. If a chemical neotoxin makes you feel ill or 'high' put 'I' or 'H' in the appropriate box. Name the brand or make of substance that makes you feel ill, e.g. brand and detergent.

Table 6.6 **Chemical neotoxin questionnaire**

Chemical Neotoxin	Never exposed	Exposed once a month	Exposed 1–3 times a wk	Exposed every day
HEATING, TRANSPORT AND OTHER FUMES				
Petrol fumes				
Diesel fumes				
Paraffin fumes				
Oil fumes				
Gas fumes				
Coal fumes				
Wood fumes				
Incinerator fumes				
Cigarette smoke				

Chemical Neotoxin	Never exposed	Exposed once a month	Exposed 1–3 times a wk	Exposed every day
DIY AND OTHER DECORATING				
Solvents				
Glues				
Paint				
Varnishes				
Cleaners				
GARDENING AND CONSTRUCTION				
Pesticides				
Insecticides				
Herbicides				
Fungicides				
Fertilizers				
Compressed board				
Plywood				
Treated timber				
GENERAL AND DOMESTIC				
Drugs				
Dyes				
Plastics				
Foam insulation				
Synthetic fibres				
Carpets				
Soaps				
Detergents				
Polishes				
Perfumes				
Aftershave				
Cosmetics				
Deodorants				
Newsprint				
Treated papers				
CFC aerosols				
Refrigerants				
MEDICAL AND DENTAL				
Anaesthetic gas				
Mercury				
Amalgams				

Chemical Neotoxin	Never exposed	Exposed once a month	Exposed 1–3 times a wk	Exposed every day
INDUSTRIAL EXPOSURE				
Sulphur dioxide				
Oxides of nitrogen				
Ozone				
Lead				
Cadmium				
Aluminium				
Alcohol				
Phenols				
Terpenes				
Formaldehyde				
Other chemicals (specify)				

Physical neotoxins

Fill in the table below to assess how often you are exposed to physical neotoxins.

Table 6.7 **Physical neotoxin questionnaire**

Physical Neotoxin	Never exposed	Exposed once a month	Exposed 1–3 times a wk	Exposed every day
TV				
VDU and computers				
Air conditioning				
HV power lines				
Hair dryers				
Mains shavers				
Electric overblankets				
Heated water beds				
Transformers				
Electric motors				

Physical Neotoxin	Never exposed	Exposed once a month	Exposed 1–3 times a wk	Exposed every day
Generators				
CB transmitters				
Radio transmitters				
TV transmitters				
Radar transmitters				
Microwave transmitters				
Mobile phones				
Microwave ovens				
Fluorescent lights				
Sunbeds				
X-rays				
Nuclear reactors				
Military bases				
Radon gas				
Jet travel				
Ultrasound scans				
Loud noises				
Geopathic stress				

Mental neotoxins

Fill in the table below to assess how often you
are exposed to mental neotoxins.

Table 6.8 **Mental neotoxin questionnaire**

Mental Neotoxin	Never exposed	Exposed once a month	Exposed 1–3 times a wk	Exposed every day
Stress at work				
Arguments at work				
Deadlines at work				

Mental Neotoxin	Never exposed	Exposed once a month	Exposed 1–3 times a wk	Exposed every day
Interruptions at work				
Excess responsibilities at work				
Frustration at work				
Work more than 10 hrs a day				
Shift work				
Changing jobs				
Unemployment				
Threat of unemployment				
Financial problems				
Family problems				
Family arguments				
Problems with children				
Police problems				
Legal problems				
Personal illness				
Illness in family				
Overcrowding				
Travelling problems				

CHECKLIST OF FACTORS THAT MAKE ALLERGIES BETTER OR WORSE

While you are carrying out the Superhealth self-assessment, you will need to become your own detective. One very useful clue that will help you to identify the neotoxin that is troubling you is to analyse the *activities, places* and *times* that make the allergy better or worse.

Paradoxically, a neotoxin can make you feel either worse *or* better. It may make you feel better due to the 'masking' effect (see page 33). You then feel worse (the withdrawal hangover), when the neotoxin is withdrawn.

Fill in Table 6.9 to find out which activities, places and times make your allergy better or

133

Table 6.9a **Activities affecting your allergy**

Please rate your 'effect on your allergy' in the appropriate column as follows:

B   = better
W = worse
NC = no change

Activities	Effect on your allergy	Comments
Sleeping		
Eating		
Drinking		
Sitting		
Standing		
Walking		
Exercising hard		
Deep breathing		
Travelling		
Smoking		
Cooking		
Cleaning		
Washing		
Hobbies		
Worrying		
Relaxing		
Any other activity (specify)		

worse than usual. During the Superhealth lifestyle change, you will be rating these factors on your environmental diary (see page 142).

It is advisable to assess the main areas in your life (job/home and hobbies/your bedroom) separately to identify your source of neotoxins.

Your job and allergies
Table 6.11 lists common jobs with their sources of neotoxins.

Table 6.9b **Times affecting your allergy**

Please rate your 'effect on your allergy' in the appropriate column as follows:

B = better
W = worse
NC = no change

Times	Effect on your allergy	Comments
Morning		
Afternoon		
Evening		
Night		
Week		
Weekend		
Work		
Holiday		
Spring		
Summer		
Autumn		
Winter		
Month (specify range)		
Wet		
Dry		
Hot		
Cold		
Before thunderstorm		

Table 6.9c **Places affecting your allergy**

Please rate your 'effect on your allergy' in the appropriate column as follows:

B = better
W = worse
NC = no change

Places	Effect on your allergy	Comments
Indoors		
Outdoors		
Work		
Shops (specify)		
Dry cleaners		
Garage		
Busy traffic		
Bus		
Train		
Car		
City		
Country		
Near grass		
Near forest		
Seaside		
Home		
Kitchen		
Bathroom		
Room with fire in		
Bedroom		
Basement		
Loft		
Other room (specify)		

To help you tie-in a specific allergen with particular places, Table 6.10 gives a list of the common sources of neotoxins in the home.

Table 6.10 **Home sources of neotoxins**

Room	Biological neotoxin	Chemical neotoxin	Physical neotoxin
Kitchen	Foods, food additives, (E numbers), bacterial and fungal toxins, pets, chlorine in tap water	Inadequate ventilation causing build up of natural gas; oven fumes (CO and NO_2), oven cleaners, washing up liquid, cleaners, soft plastics, refrigerator gases, urea formaldehyde foam insulation (UFFI), ozone/electrical devices	Large electric and magnetic fields from devices, e.g. blenders, mixers, kettles, electric stoves, fridges, dishwashers, fluorescent light, sound
Dining room (with central heating boiler)	Pets and feathers, house dust mite in carpet, pollens from indoor plants	Natural gas, oil, coal, fumes from boiler, formaldehyde and other fumes from carpet, plastics, solvents, and paints, polishes, UFFI	Electric and magnetic fields from electrical devices, TV and toasters
Living room (with open fire)	Pets and feathers, house dust mite in carpet, pollens from indoor plants	Natural gas, coal, fumes from fire, formaldehyde and other fumes from carpet, plastics, solvents, paints and polishes, UFFI	Electric and magnetic fields from fires, TV, video, sound
Bathroom	Fungi due to damp, water-borne infections chlorine in tap water	Cosmetics, antiseptics, perfumes, deodorants, formaldehyde from: shower curtains, UFFI, bleach, drain cleaners	Electric and magnetic fields from electric shavers, electric hair dryers, electrical effect of shower, radiant heaters
Washroom	Fungi due to damp, water-borne infections chlorine in tap water	Detergents, bleach, cleaners, drain cleaners, formaldehyde from plastics, solvents, paints and glues, UFFI	Electric and magnetic fields from washing machines, hot air dryer, spindryer, radiant heater
Loft	Fungi due to leaking roof, water-borne infections, dust and chlorine in roof tank. Feathers from nesting birds and dust	Pesticides from wood treatments, formaldehyde from plasters, solvents, paints and glues. UFFI, asbestos	Electric and magnetic fields from rooftop transmitters

Room	Biological neotoxin	Chemical neotoxin	Physical neotoxin
Garage and storeroom	Fungi due to damp, pets, feathers	Petrochemical fumes, solvents and glues, paints, plastics, stored pesticides, formaldehyde from stored chemicals and UFFI and ozone from electrical devices	Electric and magnetic fields from power tools for hobbies

Table 6.11 **Occupation sources of neotoxins**

Occupation	Biological neotoxin	Chemical neotoxin	Physical neotoxin (EM waves and sound)	Mental neotoxin (Stress)
Builders and construction workers	Wood dust, fungi and house dust mite	Paints, solvents, glues, formaldehyde, metals (lead, chromium and nickel), oils and tars, asbestos, pesticides	UV light (outdoor work) Noise	Heat, cold, weather, travelling, accidents
Chemical workers		Mainly the chemical manufactured plus formaldehyde, phenols, terpenes, benzene, isocyanides, halocarbons, vinyl chloride, enzymes, asbestos, gases (SO_2, Cl, NO_2, CO, NH_3, hydrocarbons), metals (Pb, As, Ni)	Electric and magnetic fields from machines, and noise	Shift work
Drivers	House dust mites in seats	Petrochemical fumes, carbon monoxide, oxides of nitrogen, formaldehyde and oils	Electric and magnetic fields from ignition Noise	Stress of being in traffic, shift work, absence from home
Electrical and electronic workers	Installation work, animal-borne disease	Aluminium, lead, bismuth, cadmium, mercury, platinum and other metals, formaldehyde, PCB, vinyl chloride, tars and oils, ozone	Strong electric and magnetic fields	Factory work: repetitive and stressful.
Farmers and agricultural workers	Animal and water-borne diseases, fungal infections, antibiotics and hormones, pollens and animal hair	Pesticides, fertilizers and many chemicals, formaldehyde, arsenic and mercury, phosphorus	Electric and magnetic fields from farm equipment Noise	Long hours

Occupation	Biological neotoxin	Chemical neotoxin	Physical neotoxin (EM waves and sound)	Mental neotoxin (Stress)
Firemen	Animal and water-borne infections, fungal infections	Very toxic fire fumes, formaldehyde, PCB dioxin, halocarbons, carbon monoxide, asbestos, arsenic and lead	Fire in radiation areas. Radiation risk Noise	Shift work, accidents
Food processing industry	Food sensitization, additives, infections and fungal toxins, antibiotics and hormones	Natural gas fumes, formaldehyde, disinfectant, pesticides, nitrates, benzene, asbestos, carbon monoxide and ethylene	Infra red oven radiation, microwave ovens, UV light Noise	Shift work, hot/cold environment
Hospital workers	Many infections from human secretions, antibiotics, hospital food	Formaldehyde, antiseptics, cleaners, drugs, antibiotics, anaesthetics, diagnostic reagents in laboratories	X-rays, radiotherapy, diagnostic radio-isotopes, NMR, diathermy, cautery, ultrasound	Shift work, emotionally charged work
Metal and foundry workers		Many metals including lead, nickel, mercury, zinc, arsenic, platinum, gases including SO_2, NO_2, and CO, formaldehyde, asbestos and tar	Heat and EM radiation from furnaces, radon from raw materials. Noise	Shift work, heat
Miners	Poor underground sanitation, animal and water-borne infections	Gases including methane, carbon monoxide, formaldehyde and phenols, metals including aluminium, arsenic, chromium, zinc, asbestos and tar	Radon, other radioactive substances and noise	Shift work, emotionally charged work. No natural light.
Office workers	House dust mite in carpets, pollens from indoor plants	Formaldehyde (many sources), solvents and glues, disinfectants and cleaners, polishes and PCB's	Static electricity, fluorescent light. Negative ion deficiency, VDU radiation, much electrical equipment	Deadlines, interruptions, telephones and meetings

Occupation	Biological neotoxin	Chemical neotoxin	Physical neotoxin (EM waves and sound)	Mental neotoxin (Stress)
Paints and plastic workers		Isocyanates, halocarbons, formaldehyde, vinyl chloride, benzene, asbestos, antimony, arsenic, chromium, lead, mercury, nickel	Electric and magnetic fields from machines, noise	Shift work
Pest control workers	Animal and water-borne infections, fungal infections	Pesticides, halocarbons, PCB, dioxin, arsenic, mercury, thallium, vanadium, formaldehyde and ethylene dibromide	UV light for insect control	
Printers		Halocarbons, solvents, glues, benzene, formaldehyde, asbestos, lead, chromium, phosphorus	Electric and magnetic fields from machines, noise	Shift work
Rubber and dye workers		Many chemicals including petrochemicals, benzene, aniline dyes, formaldehyde, halocarbons, antimony, arsenic, chromium, nickel, thallium, vanadium, zinc	Electric and magnetic fields from machines, noise	Shift work, heat
Service engineers	Animal and water-borne infections, fungal toxins	Asbestos, arsenic, formaldehyde, halocarbons, petrochemicals, lead, carbon monoxide, sulphur dioxide and ozone	Electric and magnetic fields from machines, noise	Shift work, heat/cold
Telecommunication workers		Formaldehyde, PCBs, vinyl chloride, tars and oils, ozones, metals including lead, aluminium	High levels radio and microwaves, non-ionization radiation, high level electric and magnetic fields	
Textile and clothes workers	Cotton and other fibre dusts	Formaldehyde, halocarbons, benzene, antimony and asbestos	Electric and magnetic fields from machines, noise	Shift work

Table 6.11 **Occupation sources of neotoxins**

Occupation	Biological neotoxin	Chemical neotoxin	Physical neotoxin (EM waves and sound)	Mental neotoxin (Stress)
Vehicle mechanics	House dust mite in carpets	Petrochemical fumes, carbon monoxide, nitrogen dioxide, formaldehyde, sulphur dioxide, oils, halocarbons, solvents, PCB, benzene, asbestos, ethylene glycol, ethylene dibromide, lead and chromium	Electric and magnetic fields from machines, noise	Heat/cold
VDU operators	House dust mite from carpets	Formaldehyde (many sources), solvents and glues, disinfectants and cleaners, PCB	ELF, microwaves. UV in x-rays, static electricity, fluorescent light	Stressful without proper breaks

You can analyse your own job looking for the four sources of neotoxins. List your present and previous occupations, the number of years you have carried them out, and give a brief description of the equipment and chemicals used.

Table 6.12 **Job history**

Occupation	Years worked: give approximate dates	Job description (list equipment and chemicals used)
1.		
2.		
3.		
4.		
5.		

In order to find out which neotoxin is causing your problems, you will need to keep an Environmental Diary as shown in Table 6.13.

Trigger events and your life event chart

Allergies often start following a trigger event, e.g. infection, massive exposure to chemicals or radiation, or else after a shock, accident or

Table 6.13 **Environmental Diary**

Name: .... Date.................. Weight (naked) am...................
pm...................

Time	Biological Neotoxins		Chemical Neotoxins		Physical Neotoxins	Mental Neotoxins	Pulse Rate	Symptoms 0–4	Comments
	Eating	Drinking	Activity	Place	Electrical Devices	Stress			
4.00 pm									
6.00 pm									
8.00 pm									
10.00 pm									
Midnight									
2.00 am									
4.00 am									
6.00 am									
8.00 am									
10.00 am									
Noon									
2.00 pm									
4.00 pm									

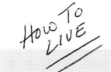

bereavement. Alternatively, allergies may be started by long term exposure to a provocant, often at a concentration below the presently accepted danger level, e.g. petrochemical fumes. In order to decide if you may be at risk fill in a Life Event Chart similar to the one below, listing:

- when you were completely well (mark with a tick);
- when any symptoms commenced (mark with a cross);
- a correlation of your symptoms with infections, chemical exposure, job, housing, hobbies and social situation

The CADTEMP (Computer Aided Diagnosis and Treatment of Environmental Medical Problems), produces a Life Event Chart from your answers to standard questions.

THE SUPERHEALTH LIFESTYLE CHANGE

After you have filled in the Superhealth self-assessment questionnaire, you should have a good idea of the neotoxins to which you are over exposed.

You will need to follow the relevant chapters in the book to decide an individual sus-ceptibility, but this section will tell you how to reduce your total load of neotoxins.

How do I reduce my total load of biological neotoxins?

Organic food

Eat only organic food (i.e. nothing that has been sprayed with chemicals or pesticides). You can be happy that it is organic if it has the imprint of the Soil Association. Try to avoid anything from a packet, tin or bottle, especially if it contains any E numbers.

Table 6 **Life Event Chart**

Date	Infection	Chemical exposure	House type	Jobs	Hobbies	Social changes	Symptoms
1980 ✓				Nurse	Gardening	Father died	
1981 X	Dysentery						Colitis
1982			17th century cottage	VDU operator		Changed job	
1983 X		Chemical spill at work					Depression
1984						Marriage	
1985							
1986 X			Flat (built 1986)			Moved house	Persistently tired
1987	Meningitis				DIY	Promotion	
1988						Mother died	
1989 X						Pregnancy	Migraine
1990						Left work	
1991						Second pregnancy	

Bottled water

Drink and cook with bottled water only, preferably from glass bottles. Drink at least 3 pints of fluid a day as this will help to flush out poisons from your body.

Food preparation

Prepare your food properly and be careful not to handle cooked and uncooked meats with the same utensils. Cook thoroughly and avoid the use of microwave ovens.

Pets and pollens

If you are allergic to your pets or flowers, try to keep them out of the house as much as possible. Even if you are not allergic, make sure you keep pets and pollens out of your bedroom (you sleep in there for 8 hours).

Hay fever

If you have hay fever, keep your windows closed during the day in the hay fever season. You may open them briefly after heavy rainstorms, when pollen levels are greatly reduced.

Damp and fungi

Keep your house dry, especially your bedroom. Damp encourages growth of fungi and house dust mites.

House dust mite

If you are allergic to house dust mites (i.e. you suffer from rhinitis, runny eyes or asthma which is worse in bed), then follow the measures described on page 166 to remove house dust mite.

Infections

Take all reasonable steps to avoid all sources of infections.

How do I reduce my total load of chemical neotoxins?

Reduce your total load of chemical neotoxins at home by the following methods.

HOUSE

Correct site for your house

First, find the direction of the prevailing wind. Then avoid being near or downwind of industrial areas, factories, chemical dumps, busy roads, especially junctions (or agricultural land that is sprayed). People allergic to trees or grass pollens should also avoid woods and fields. A house site needs to be well drained to avoid damp which causes the growth of fungi. Don't live in a house built on a landfill site since these give off methane, and highly toxic chemicals may have been dumped there. *NO*

Construction

Modern house construction methods release a very wide range of chemicals. Urea Formaldehyde Foam Insulation (UFFI) in cavity walls is now banned in Canada. Any house with this form of insulation is totally unsatisfactory, since the UFFI continues to release formaldehyde into the house for years after the installation. Wide use of formaldehyde-releasing woods, boards, plastics, glues and paints is also unacceptable. Asbestos should also be avoided since it raises the risk of cancer. Recent spraying with antifungals (e.g. Pentachlorophenol) is also very dangerous.

Furnishings and decorations

Remove as many synthetic materials, including fabrics, foams, carpets, curtains, plywoods, block board and plastics as possible. Replace these with metal, glass, unbleached natural fibres and bare wood or tiles.

Heating

Review the heating system of the house. Try to replace natural gas with electricity (unless you are electrically sensitive). If you have a boiler try to have it sited in a sealed room which does not communicate with the rest of the house. Make sure the chimneys and flues remove the exhaust gases fully so that they do not leak back into the house.

Cooking

Consider changing your natural gas cooker to an electric one. If you decide to change your gas cooker you should also have all the old gas pipes removed. Unused gas pipes will still continue to leak tiny amounts of gas. Replace your teflon and aluminium cooking utensils with glass and stainless steel.

Ventilation

Increase the ventilation through the house, especially in the kitchen and bedroom, by installing extractor fans.

Clothing

Wear only natural unbleached fibres coloured with natural dyes. Try to make sure that fibres have not been treated with pesticides for moth proofing.

Aerosols and beauty products

Completely avoid aerosols since the pro-pellants are the highly allergic fluorinated hydrocarbons (CFCs). Also try to avoid using cosmetics, deodorants and other beauty products, since they often cause problems.

Washing

When washing your body, use only plain soap without perfume. When washing your clothes use a non-biological detergent. After washing, rinse your clothes with an extra washing cycle without powder.

Storage

Don't store bleaches, cleaners, disinfectants and polishes in parts of the house that you frequently use. Start using less chemically active substances for these purposes. Fortunately the green movement is providing alternatives which are much less toxic to the environment and to humans. It is not necessary to 'kill all known germs', so use these materials very sparingly.

Garage

If you have an integral garage, don't park your car in there because fumes will come into the house and especially into the room above the garage.

Smoking

Give up smoking. If you don't smoke but somebody else in the house is a smoker, do your best to persuade them not to smoke indoors. Otherwise try to get them to restrict their smoking to rooms that you don't use.

Sleeping

You spend 8 hours a day in your bedroom. However, unfortunately, the average bedroom is filled with many possible sources of chemical sensitivity. Even if you don't change any other part of your house, convert your bedroom to a chemically clean area. Consider using a small room for a bedroom, and adapt it as follows:

- Move everything non-essential out;
- Remove all the synthetic fabrics, foams, carpets and plastics, and replace them with non-bleached cotton and wool bedding and metal and glass fittings;
- Try to store your clothes, books and other possessions somewhere else, since they tend to give off formaldehyde.

How do I reduce my total load of chemical neotoxins in the office?

Reduce your total load of chemical neotoxins in the office by the following methods:

Choice of office

If you have the choice, avoid a modern air-conditioned office with no opening windows. These frequently cause illnesses.

Avoid solvents

Try to avoid all solvents. Stop using marker pens, liquid typewriter correcting fluid and synthetic glues.

Photocopying machines

Try to make sure that the photocopying machine is located in a well ventilated spot away from the work area.

Avoid polishes and cleaners

Try to avoid excessive use of polishes, waxes, carpet cleaners, air fresheners, antiseptics and fly and insect sprays.

No smoking

Encourage the office to have a no smoking policy.

Turn off electrical devices

Turn off all electrical devices when they are not in use. These give off many fumes and in addition, an increasing number of people are electrically sensitive.

How do I reduce my load of neotoxins in the factory?

Reduce your total load of chemical neotoxins in your factory by the following methods.

Protective clothing

Wear all the protective clothing provided for the job. The Health and Safety Executive is a government body with wide powers and can advise on current safety equipment *which must be provided for your use by law.*

However, chemical sensitivities occur at concentrations of chemicals far below the present 'safe' level. If you are chemically sensitive, then you may decide to find alternative employment rather than continually making yourself ill.

Activated carbon filter mask

Wear an activated carbon filter mask. This will extract a large number of chemical neotoxins from the air that you breathe. This mask must fit tightly and must be renewed regularly.

Ventilation

Ensure that there is good ventilation and circulation of fresh clean air in your work area. Check all flues, chimneys and air ducts.

Avoid solvents

Use all volatile and airborne substances, e.g. solvents, paints, glues, either outdoors or in special areas designed for their use. Wear protective masks.

No smoking

Do not smoke. Encourage the factory to have a no-smoking policy.

How can I reduce my total load of physical neotoxins?

Reduce your total load of physical neotoxins by the following methods.

Avoid EM radiation

Try not to live or work near a high voltage power line, electric motor, generator or transformer, transmitter, nuclear reactor or reprocessing plant, or military installations.

Reduce exposure to VDUs

Reduce your exposure to electric and magnetic fields by turning off all devices when not in use, e.g. turn off VDUs and don't use them for more than 4 hours a day, or more than an hour at a time without a break.

High risk electrical devices

Completely avoid using electric overblankets, heated water beds, sunbeds and microwave ovens.

X-rays and conception

Don't have any unnecessary x-ray investigations, especially in the 3 months before conception of a child. This rule applies to men *and* women.

Reduce noise level

Reduce your work and home sound level so that you can easily hold a conversation in a normal speaking voice.

Reduce geopathic stress

Review your sleeping place to see if it may be subject to geopathic stress.

How can I reduce my total load of mental neotoxins?

Reduce your total load of mental neotoxins by the following methods.

Have reasonable objectives

Decide on a very few well-defined reasonable objectives and don't take on too many tasks.

Have a positive response to stress

Change your response to stress. Always try to be positive and constructive but also learn from your mistakes and don't worry too much.

Use relaxation techniques

Use relaxation techniques to cope with stress. Make sure that you get enough daily exercise and sleep. Natural relaxation and sex are also very helpful as is a strong relationship with another person.

No instant solution

Avoid 'instant' twentieth-century remedies to produce relaxation such as tranquillizers, TV, cigarettes and alcohol. Remember, there *are* no short-cuts!

How can I easily change my lifestyle to include more exercise?

The twentieth-century lifestyle actually makes it quite difficult to exercise. Insufficient attention and resources are devoted to helping people to make exercise part of their lives. Exercise for adults is often seen as a television spectator sport!

Your Superhealth lifestyle change should include physical exercise and mental relaxation. It will do this in two ways:

- By identifying changes that you can make in your lifestyle so that you are able to increase the exercise content of your day with only a little extra effort.
- By helping you plan a thirty minute vigorous session twice or three times a week at an activity you enjoy.

A personal fitness plan is not a new idea, and in fact it was quite usual for the ancient Greeks to consult both a physician and a trainer in order to recover from illness. The former would diagnose and treat ailments, and the latter would work out a customized series of exercises and activities to get the patient back to fitness and health.

The Superhealth Exercise Tips

- Don't ride when you can walk.
- Park your car, or get off the bus several stops before your destination, and walk the remaining distance.

- Change your route so you can walk or run through the park (in daylight) on the way to work.
- Use the stairs, not the lift. If it is a skyscraper, get out four floors before your destination and walk the last four floors (your colleagues will be very impressed). If you are feeling a little less energetic, go four floors above your destination and walk down: it is still exercise. Do the same when leaving.
- Don't do everything by telephone. Make a personal visit sometimes. The exercise and face-to-face contact will help you work more efficiently.
- Buy a bicycle to ride to work. However, don't ride it in smog-filled underpasses or in the rain or snow, when cycling is often dangerous.
- Use exercise as a substitute for other things you are cutting out of your life, such as cigarettes, alcohol, food.
- Use exercise as part of your stress management programme.

How do vitamins and minerals deficiencies occur?

Adequate amounts of vitamins, minerals and other nutrients are essential for good health. They are particularly important in allergic disease, since they help the body to repair itself. During an allergic illness the daily requirement of a specific vitamin, mineral or other nutrient may be dramatically increased.

Deficiencies of vitamins, minerals and other nutrients may occur because of several reasons.

Inadequate dietary intake for the state of health

Allergic and ill people need more vitamins and minerals. The Recommended Daily Allowance (RDA) which is so often quoted is the minimum amount needed by fit people to stop deficiency disease. This is not a meaningful figure, since the amount required for *optimum* health is usually considerably higher, especially in an ill person.

Interaction of vitamins, minerals and other substances and bacteria in the gut

Despite having an adequate dietary intake, a deficiency may arise due to interaction of vitamins and minerals with other substances found in the gut (e.g., vitamin D being bound to phytic acid in flour). The bacteria normally living in the bowel can be altered after a course of antibiotics and then the altered bacteria may destroy vitamins.

A failure of absorption of the vitamins, minerals and other nutrients

If the bowel is damaged physically or biochemically it is unable to absorb vitamins and minerals properly. Physical damage occurs in coeliac disease when the convoluted high surface area small bowel is replaced with a flat, lower surface area bowel. Biochemical damage occurs after infection or poisoning, at which time enzyme damage occurs, and active absorption is greatly reduced.

Failure of utilization

After vitamins and minerals are absorbed they enter the circulation. However, sometimes they cannot be used properly, due to a deficiency of another substance. For example adequate levels of Vitamin B_{12} cannot be used unless folic acid is also present in sufficient amounts.

How can I ensure that I get adequate vitamins and minerals?

- Have a varied diet, don't eat the same thing every day. Instead, rotate food families (see page 233) and occasionally stop eating a popular food for three days.

- Buy fresh food and eat soon after purchase. Vitamin content is reduced by light, and storage at room temperature. Refrigeration, cooling and dark storage all reduce the rate of vitamin loss.
- Where possible, cook and eat fruit and vegetables with the skin on, as the vitamin content is much higher. However, chemicals penetrate sprayed (non-organic) fruit, and if the skin is eaten, high levels of poison may be absorbed.
- When preparing and cooking food, avoid prolonged soaking or cooking because this reduces vitamin content.
- Cook your food in bottled water. Tap water often contains unacceptable contaminants.
- Eat food immediately after cooking. Standing reduces vitamin content.

Vitamin and mineral deficiencies are quite common in the western world, due to the low vitamin and mineral content of food, and to the increased requirements secondary to stress, pollution and allergies.

Most people need vitamin and mineral supplements. The exact dose should be tailored to your individual requirements, e.g. for children, men, women (pregnant, breast feeding), in sickness or in health.

It is important to remember that, although the body is able to synthesize some of the vitamins, it cannot make any mineral. Consequently, it is essential that these are taken either in the diet or as a supplement.

When you are taking vitamins and minerals, try to follow these guidelines:

- Make sure there are no additives, colours or flavours in the mineral or vitamin

Table 6.15 **Typical daily vitamin supplement for adults**

A	5,000 iu	
B₁	50 mg	B complex vitamins. The 'anti-stress' vitamins should be taken together rather than singly
B₂	50 mg	
B₃	50 mg	
B₅	100 mg	
B₆	50 mg	
C	2,000 mg	The 'anti-pollution' vitamin
E	200 iu	The 'anti-oxidant' vitamin
Calcium	500 mg	Taken as Dolomite tablet
Magnesium	250 mg	The 'anti-stress' mineral. Take as Dolomite tablet
Zinc	15 mg	Take as chelated zinc if possible
Evening Primrose Oil	1,500 mg	Source of essential Omega 6 fatty acids

NB The daily dosage of vitamins and minerals will need to be increased during pregnancy and breast feeding. The doses for children are considerably less than the adult dose. Ideally, vitamin intake should be supervised by a suitably qualified person and tailored to each individual's requirements.

supplement. Check that you are not allergic to the filler, e.g. lactose (milk sugar), or cornflour which makes up the bulk of the tablet.

- Take 'chelated' mineral tablets if available. A 'chelated' mineral is more easily absorbed. Non-chelated minerals are less well absorbed, especially in ill patients, and the dose received is far less.
- Vitamins and minerals reduce the effectiveness of antibiotics. If you are taking antibiotics, take your supplement one hour before or two hours after the antibiotic.
- Take vitamins that come from natural sources rather than synthetically produced ones. Although the vitamins from both sources are chemically identical, the other substances found with the naturally occurring vitamins make it more effective and less likely to cause side effects.

How can I tell if I have a vitamin or mineral deficiency?

Unfortunately, there is no easy way to tell if you have a vitamin or mineral deficiency.

Tables 6.16 and 6.17 list some of the major deficiency symptoms. However, many of these have a gradual onset and are very similar to allergic symptoms. If you take the vitamin supplements as advised, you are much less likely to be deficient.

Mineral deficiencies in contrast, can be confirmed by carrying out a hair analysis. Hair analysis laboratories are listed in the 'Useful Addresses' in the appendix. It is essential to have your results interpreted by an expert to understand the full significance of the test. Some mineral deficiencies can suggest the presence of diseases, e.g. low calcium, magnesium and elevated sodium and potassium may suggest cystic fibrosis. The technique of hair analysis is also able to show the presence of toxic metals such as mercury, aluminium, arsenic and cadmium.

Tables 6.16 and 6.17 list the important vitamins, minerals and other nutrients. Rich sources of the vitamin/mineral are listed as are the use to which they are put in the body. Symptoms of deficiency are listed together with relevant comments.

Table 6.16 **Vitamins, their sources and effects**

Vitamin	Rich sources of vitamin	Used by the body for: Deficiencies cause	Comments
A (fat soluble anti-oxidant)	Oily fish (e.g. herrings and tuna) and fish oils, egg yolk, dairy products, yellow/orange vegetables (e.g. carrots)	Vitamin A maintains mucous membrane in the mouth and bowel, eyes and nose. It is also needed for red blood cell and hormone formation. Deficiency causes ulcers of the mucous membranes and an increased susceptibility to infection	Vitamin A level is reduced by raised fat and mineral oils, air pollution, alcohol, steroids and aspirin

Vitamin	Rich sources of vitamin	Used by the body for: Deficiencies cause	Comments
D (fat soluble)	Sunshine (reacts with oils in skin to form Vit.D). Fish oils, oily fish, dairy products, eggs	Vitamin D is needed for calcium, metabolism, growth and maintenance of bones and teeth. Deficiency can cause symptoms similar to female menopause, i.e. hot flushes, sweats, depression, irritability, nervousness, cramp and soft bones	Overdose of Vitamin D can cause calcification in kidneys. High dose of Vit.D contraindicated with digoxin. Vit.D is reduced by alcohol, steroids and oral contraceptive
E (fat soluble anti-oxidant)	Unrefined cold pressed oils, whole grains, dairy products, egg yolk, nuts, pulses and green vegetables	Vitamin E is the antioxidant vitamin that removes dangerous 'free radicals' from the body that may cause allergies. It also prevents destruction of Vit.A. Deficiency of Vit.E causes anorexia, premature ageing and infertility. Vitamin E, despite being fat soluble, is not stored	Vitamin E should be used with care with hyperthyroidism, raised blood pressure or rheumatoid arthritis. Vit.E level is reduced by chemical neotoxins, antibiotics, chlorine, iron, minerals and oral contraceptive and rancid fat
B_1 Thiamin (water soluble)	Whole grains, offal, brewers yeast, pulses, nuts and eggs	Vitamin B_1 is required to convert glucose to energy or fat and for healthy nerves and muscles. Deficiency causes many allergic-like symptoms including weakness, fatigue, depression, insomnia, headaches, aching and stiffness, back pains, indigestion and flatulence, palpitations and shortness of breath	B Vitamins need to be taken together. They are less effective taken singly. Deficiency tends to cause mental symptoms first. Vit.B_1 is destroyed by alcohol, antibiotics and excess sugar in the diet
B_2 Riboflavin (water soluble)	Brewers yeast, whole grains, green vegetables, dairy products, egg, pulses and offal	Vitamin B_2 is needed for metabolism of carbohydrates, fats and proteins. Deficiency causes sensitivity to light, sore and bloodshot eyes, cheeks with many small blister marks, dry peeling lips. Many alcoholics have B_2 deficiencies	Vit.B_2 is destroyed by alcohol, antibiotics, and oral contraceptives, and ultra violet light

Vitamin	Rich sources of vitamin	Used by the body for: Deficiencies cause	Comments
B_3 Nicotinamide or Niacin (water soluble)	Brewers yeast, whole grains, fish, poultry, nuts, offal	Vitamin B_3 is required directly or indirectly for most body processes including metabolism of carbohydrates, fat and proteins. Deficiency produces dermatitis, diarrhoea and dementia (the 3 'D's). It may also cause depression, tension, insomnia and impaired memory	Vit.B_3 is destroyed by alcohol, antibiotics and excess dietary sugar. It should be used with care in people with severe diabetes, glaucoma, peptic ulcer or reduced liver function
B_5 Pantothenic acid (water soluble)	Brewers yeast, whole grains, green vegetables, pulses, offal, poultry and fish	Vitamin B_5 is required for the metabolism and release of energy from fat and carbo-hydrates. Deficiency stops the adrenal working properly and causes low blood pressure and blood sugar, also fatigue, weakens muscle and joints, causes aches, palpitations and depression	Vitamin B_5 is destroyed by aspirin and methyl bromide (an insecticide fumigant)
B_6 Pyridoxine (water soluble)	Brewers yeast, whole grains, offal and eggs	Vitamin B_6 is needed to process magnesium, zinc and manganese, Essential Fatty Acids (EFA) and many amino acids (building blocks for proteins). Defiency of B_6 can cause a very wide variety of allergy-like symptoms including headache, irritability, nervousness, inability to concentrate, lethargy, anorexia, abdomen pains, nausea and vomiting, diarrhoea, haemorrhoids and cracked skin	Vitamin B_6 needs to be taken with B vitamins especially B_2, zinc and magnesium. B_6 should not be taken with anti-parkinsonian drugs such as levadopa. Vitamin B_6 is destroyed by alcohol, smoking, steroids, oral contraceptive and oestrogen
B_{12} Cyanocobalamin (water soluble)	Dairy products, red meat and eggs, offal, fish	Vitamin B_{12} is needed to make and maintain cell membranes. Deficiency causes pernicious anaemia, damage to nerves, sore mouth and tongue	Vitamin B_{12} is obtained almost exclusively from animal products. Con-sequently vegetarians need to take ade-quate supplements. Increased B_{12} is required with high dose of Vit.C. Vit.B_{12} must always be given with adequate folic

Vitamin	Rich sources of vitamin	Used by the body for: Deficiencies cause	Comments
			acid because a relative deficiency of the latter could cause pernicious anaemia
Folic Acid (member of B complex) (water soluble)	Deep green leafy vegetables, carrots, brewers yeast, whole grains	Needed for cell division and metabolism of sugar and amino acids, formation of blood and antibodies. Deficiency can cause pernicious anaemia, depression, fatigue and susceptibility to infection	Increased doses of folic acid are needed by people under stress and on high doses of Vit.C, growing children and pregnant women. Excess of folic acid can precipitate pernicious anaemia in people who are relatively deficient in Vitamin B_{12}. Folic acid can reduce the effects of sulphonamides and anti-convulsants. Folic acid is destroyed by alcohol, anti-convulsants, oral contraceptive and barbiturates
Biotin (B complex) (water soluble)	Brewers yeast, nuts, offal, egg yolk, brown rice, pulses and dark green vegetables	Biotin is necessary for fat and protein metabolism. Deficiency causes depression, fatigue, muscular pain, panic attacks, dry peeling skin and hair loss	Biotin is destroyed by antibiotics, sulphonamides, and egg white (albumen)
Choline (B complex) (fat soluble)	Egg yolk, offal, green leafy vegetables, Brewers yeast, whole grains	Needed for formation of DNA and RNA, muscle and nerve function, memory and manganese metabolism. Deficiency may cause headaches, dizziness and high blood pressure	Choline is destroyed by insecticides, alcohol, sulphon-amides, the oral contraceptive pill, oestrogen and excess dietary sugar

Table 6.16 **Vitamins, their sources and effects**

Vitamin	Rich sources of vitamin	Used by the body for: Deficiencies cause	Comments
C Ascorbic Acid (anti-oxidant) (water soluble)	Citrus fruits, rosehips, berries, green and leafy vegetables, tomatoes and potatoes	Vitamin C detoxifies pollutants. It is needed to remove the free-radicals caused by neotoxins. It keeps the skin, bones, muscles healthy and promotes healing after infection, injury and surgery. Deficiency causes many allergic–like symptoms including fatigue, irritability, depression, weakness, muscle and joint pains, gum and skin damage	Vitamin C is destroyed by a very wide range of substances including alcohol, antibiotics, antihistamines, aspirin, barbiturates, insecticides, oral contraceptive, oestrogen, petrochemicals, smoking

Table 6.17 **Minerals, their sources and effects**

Mineral	Rich sources of mineral	Used by the body for: Deficiencies cause	Comments
Calcium	Dairy products, pulses, offal, fish, green vegetables, egg	Calcium is necessary for nerve and muscle function, blood clotting, bones and teeth. Deficiency causes many allergy-like symptoms including irritability, insomnia, palpitations, constipation, PMT, long-term lack causes rickets, osteoporosis and even fractures	Calcium is lost during bed rest and high protein diets. Calcium is lost by the action of steroids and aspirin, and excess phosphorus
Magnesium	Figs, citrus fruits, nuts, dark green vegetables	Magnesium is needed for energy production, function of nerves, muscles and many enzymes, and protein synthesis. Deficiency causes tremors and twitching, palpitations and cramp. Mental symptoms include depression, poor memory, increased sensitivity to noise and hyper-sensitivity in children	Magnesium and calcium metabolism are interelated especially in the blood stream. Deficiency or excess of one causes problems with the other. Magnesium is lost by the action of alcohol, steroids and diuretics (water tablets)

Mineral	Rich sources of mineral	Used by the body for: Deficiencies cause	Comments
Phosphorus	Fish, poultry, meat, whole grains, eggs, seeds and nuts	Phosphorous is needed for most intracellular reactions including growth, repair, and production of energy. Deficiency is rare because most foods contain phosphorus	Calcium and Vit.D are essential for proper phosphorus metabolism. Phosphorus is lost by the action of alcohol antacids, aspirin, diuretics and steroids
Potassium	Citrus fruits, all green leafy vegetables, bananas and potatoes	Potassium is needed for function of nerves and muscles. Deficiency causes weakness, irritability, diarrhoea, constipation and cramp	Potassium may be lost by the action of aspirin, diuretics, sodium chloride (common salt) and steroids
Iron	Red meat, offal, eggs, whole grains, shellfish, dried fruit	Iron is needed to make haemoglobin present as the oxygen carrying pigment in red blood cells. Deficiency causes anaemia which causes weakness, shortness of breath, palpitations, fatigue, depression, mental confusion and poor memory. Iron deficiency is much more common in women	Iron is much better absorbed with Vit.C. Iron should *not* be given to anyone suffering from sickle cell anaemia, thallassaemia or haemochromatosis. Iron is lost by the effect of antacids, aspirin, anti-inflammatory pain killers, EDTA (a food preservative)
Zinc	Red meat, whole grains, brewers yeast, offal	Zinc is needed for the formation of many enzymes and control of protein synthesis, contraction of muscles, formation of insulin, and fertility. Zinc deficiency causes white spots on fingernails, stretch marks on skin, poor hair growth, acne, period problems, infertility, arthritis and cold extremeties	Zinc deficiency is very common in developed countries. Iron supplements interfere with zinc absorption and these two minerals should be taken on alternate days. Zinc supplements should be taken with Vit.A. Zinc is lost due to the effect of alcohol, diuretics, oral contraceptive and steroids.

Mineral	Rich sources of mineral	Used by the body for: Deficiencies cause	Comments
Copper	Whole grains, pulses, offal and seafood	Copper is necessary for the use of Vit.C, iron and amino acids. Deficiency causes anaemia and oedema	Excess copper is toxic
Manganese	Nuts, green leafy vegetables, whole grains, pulses, egg yolks	Manganese activates many enzymes including those used for digestion, utilization of food bone growth and reproduction. Deficiency causes fatigue, irritability and memory loss.	Manganese uptake is reduced in the presence of insecticides. Hyperactive children and epileptics often have low manganese. This mineral is lost due to the effect of antibiotics
Selenium (the anti-oxidant mineral)	Whole grains, tuna fish, onions, tomatoes, broccoli	Selenium neutralizes 'free radicals' which otherwise would cause tissue damage and diseases. Selenium stops ageing. Deficiency causes muscular weakness and infertility	Selenium works particularly well in the presence of Vit.E. Men have a greater need for selenium than women
Chromium	Red meat, shellfish, chicken, whole grains, brewers yeast	Chromium is needed for sugar and protein metabolism. Deficiency may cause high blood pressure and encourage the onset of diabetes	Chelated zinc may sometimes help in chromium deficiency
Nickel	Whole grains, vegetables	Nickel is an activator of some enzymes. It is also needed for hormone production and cell membrane metabolism. Deficiency aggravates iron-deficiency anaemia	Nickel toxicity or sensitization can occur due to industrial exposure. Cigarette smoke contains nickel
Cobalt	Red meat, offal, shellfish	Cobalt is necessary for sugar metabolism and formation of blood cells and nerves. Deficiency causes pernicious anaemia	Vegetarians may suffer cobalt deficiency without a B_{12} supplement. Cobalt is lost due to the effect of oral contraceptives

Table 6.18 **Other Nutrients**

Other nutrients	Rich sources of mineral	Used by the body for: Deficiencies cause	Comments
Omega-3 Essential fatty acid, Eicosapentaenoic acid	Fish oils, especially herring, mackerel, salmon and tuna	Cell membrane maintenance, fat metabolism and reducing inflammation	Helpful in a very wide variety of conditions including arthritis, asthma and arterial disease
Fish Omega-6 Essential fatty acids (three types: Linoleic, Linolenic and Arachidonic acid)	Unrefined cold pressed oils, nuts, green leafy vegetables, seeds and nuts	Essential fatty acids are used by the body to produce and maintain all cell membranes, nerves and brain, hormones and prostaglandins. They are essential for absorption of fat soluble vitamins (A, D and E) and to promote growth of bacteria that usually grow in the bowel. The prostaglandin E_1 reduces inflammation and helps the immune system. Deficiency of essential fatty acids cause immune system problems, dry hair and skin, arthritis and infertility	Gamma Linolenic acid (Evening Primrose Oil) is rapidly converted to Prostaglandin E_1 in the body. It has a remarkable helpful effect in a very wide variety of conditions including eczema, arthritis, hyperactivity in children, PMT and alcoholism
Essential amino acids (8)	Animal protein in meats, dairy products, poultry, eggs, seafood. Single plant protein sources do not contain all the essential amino acids	Amino acids are the building blocks that make up proteins. The eight essential amino acids cannot be manufactured by the body but must be contained in the diet. Deficiency causes depression, fatigue, poor weight gain and reduced efficiency of the immune system	The 8 essential amino acids are isoleucine, leucine, lysine, methionine, phenylalanine, threonine, tryptophan, valine. An extra amino acid, histidine, is required by infants and children.

SUMMARY

By following 'The Superhealth Plan' of neotoxins in your life and when you remove them, achieve a big improvement in your health and energy level. By greatly reducing your total load of neotoxins you have removed a great burden from your liver, kidneys, brain, heart and lungs. Consequently, all these organs will work much better.

It is important to *change your lifestyle permanently*, otherwise you will soon return to your previous state of reduced health. Be prepared to make a major alteration to your lifestyle; in order to get a long-term improvement in health and the quality of your life you may need to make one or more personal alterations to your life style, including:

- diet change
- job change
- house move
- change your hobby
- change your social life.

The three basic rules that you should try to follow for the rest of your life are:

1. *REDUCE YOUR TOTAL LOAD OF NEOTOXINS*
2. *REDUCE PARTICULARLY THE NEO-TOXIN TO WHICH YOU ARE ESPECIALLY SENSITIVE.*
3. *USE SLEEP, REST, EXERCISE, VITAMINS, MINERALS AND OTHER SUPPLEMENTS TO HELP YOURSELF BACK TO COMPLETE HEALTH.*

PART II

HOW
ENVIRONMENTAL
MEDICINE
BEATS
ILLNESS

CHAPTER SEVEN

BEATING ASTHMA, RHINITIS, HAY FEVER AND ECZEMA

ASTHMA

Asthma has the dubious qualification of being the only major cause of childhood death that is still increasing in frequency. It is a very common disease, affecting 1 child in 10, with 1 person in 3 suffering from asthma at some time in their life.

Why is asthma becoming more common?

Asthma is becoming more common due to the general rise in neotoxins in polluted air, food and water produced by our modern style of living. The number of asthmatics in the rural third world, in contrast, is very low. The sources of neotoxins causing the increase in asthma include:

- **Biological neotoxins**
  The house dust mite has become more common in people's homes. This is due to the rise in humidity in the home produced by modern construction methods, lack of ventilation, and central heating. Fitted carpets also provide an ideal place for the house dust mite to live.

  The level of additives and other chemicals deliberately added to food is now so high that it is difficult to eat a diet free of such substances.

  Increased population densities and 'air

conditioning' systems make the incidence and spread of virus infections more common.

- **Chemical neotoxins**
  The increased level of chemical pollutants, e.g. formaldehyde, pesticides, sulphur dioxide, carbon monoxide, nitrogen dioxide, petrochemical fumes and ozone.
- **Physical neotoxins**
  The 'electric smog' coming from devices and machines at home and work.
- **Mental neotoxins**
  The high stress level that is an integral part of the twentieth century way of life.

What is asthma?

Asthma is a variable wheeze associated with breathlessness. It is caused by three processes, which together reduce the flow of air into and out of the lungs (see Figure 7.1):

- plugging of the air tubes with mucus;
- inflammation and swelling of the lining of the air tubes;
- spasm of the muscle of the air tubes.

How can I tell if I have asthma?

You are likely to develop some (though not all) of the following symptoms.

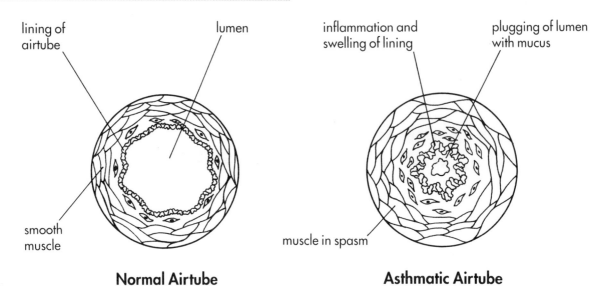

Figure 7.1 **Cross section through normal and asthmatic air tube**

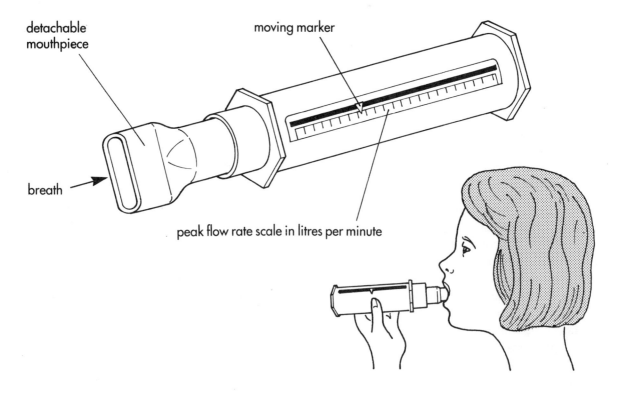

Figure 7.2 **Peak flow meter**

- dry cough ⎫ worse at night;
- wheezing, worse on ⎬ very disturbed
  breathing out ⎭ sleep;
- chest tightness on awakening, or in a cold smoky atmosphere;
- excessive shortness of breath on exertion;
- recurrent chest infections.

These symptoms are very common, and asthma is greatly underdiagnosed.

There is an objective measurement of asthma, which involves using a peak flow meter (see Figure 7.2). In the UK these may now be obtained on NHS prescription through your GP. With this instrument you can compare your own peak flow level with the predicted level for your age and height. If your peak flow is substantially reduced at rest, or if it drops by more than 15% after exercise, then you probably have asthma.

It is important to carry out the peak flow measurements properly. Do it as follows:

- Take a deep breath in;
- Hold your breath for 2 to 3 seconds;
- Put your lips around the mouth piece;
- Blow as hard as you can;
- Read the value;
- Repeat twice, choose the best figure of the three readings, and compare it with the predicted value on the Tables 7.1(a), (b) and (c).

Table 7.1(a) **Peak flow rate for children — boys and girls (predicted values)**

Height (ft & ins) (metres)	3'0" 0.91m	3'3" 0.99m	3'6" 1.07m	3'9" 1.14m	4'2" 1.22m	4'0" 1.27m	4'4" 1.32m	4'6" 1.37m	4'8" 1.42m	4'10" 1.47m	5'0" 1.52m	5'2" 1.57m
Predicted Peak Flow l/min	95	120	145	175	210	235	260	285	310	335	360	385
Abnormal if Peak Flow below	75	95	115	140	170	190	200	230	250	270	290	310

A peak flow rate of more than 20% below the predicted rate is abnormal

---

Table 7.1(b) **Peak flow rate for adult men (predicted values)**

Age	Height 5'3" (1.6m)	Height 5'6" (1.68m)	Height 5'9" (1.75m)	Height 6'0" (1.83m)	Height 6'3" (1.91m)
15 years	520	530	540	550	560
25 years	600	610	620	630	645
35 years	615	625	635	645	655

Age	Height 5'3" (1.6m)	Height 5'6" (1.68m)	Height 5'9" (1.75m)	Height 6'0" (1.83m)	Height 6'3" (1.91m)
45 years	590	605	615	625	635
55 years	565	575	590	600	610
65 years	545	555	565	580	590
70 years	535	545	555	570	580

A peak flow rate of more than 100 l/min below the predicted rate is abnormal

Table 7.1(c) **Peak flow rate for adult women (predicted values)**

Age	Height 4'9" (1.45m)	Height 5'0" (1.52m)	Height 5'3" (1.60m)	Height 5'6" (1.68m)	Height 5'9" (1.75m)
15 years	440	450	460	470	480
25 years	450	460	470	480	490
35 years	450	465	475	485	495
45 years	445	455	465	475	490
55 years	425	435	450	460	470
65 years	400	410	420	435	445
70 years	385	395	405	415	430

A peak flow rate of more than 85 l/min below the predicted rate is abnormal

Why does asthma occur?

The reason that an asthmatic attack occurs can be summarized as:

Irritable lung airways + Trigger factor (e.g. house dust mite) ——► Asthma attack

An asthmatic has unstable airways, i.e. they are more likely to go into spasm than the airways of a non-asthmatic. An asthmatic's airways remain the usual size until a trigger factor, like pollen, causes them to secrete mucus, swell up and go into spasm; i.e., an asthma attack. An asthma attack tends to start as a cough, which becomes a wheeze, and then a full blown attack.

Factors that make the lung airways more irritable include:

- **Genetic factors:** a gene has now been identified which predisposes to asthma.
- **Nocturnal variation:** the lung airways are always less able to pass air at night. This tendency is exaggerated in asthmatics.
- **Exercise:**
- **Temperature changes:** The body's unconscious responses to these changes are governed by sympathetic and parasympathetic nervous system (the autonomic system)
- **Other allergic conditions:** e.g eczema. These alter the immune system and

increase the likelihood of an asthma attack.

Trigger factors for asthmatic attacks include:

- pollens, house dust mites, birds' feathers, insects, animal furs, fungal spores, mouldy hay and other plants with fungal infections, grain dust, wood dust, cotton fibres.
- infections, (bacterial, viral, fungal and parasites).

} biological neotoxins

- Isocyanates in paints, epoxy resins, enzymes in washing powders, antibiotics and other drugs, metals and their salts, solder fumes, dyes, plastics, irritant gases e.g. formaldehyde, chlorine, tobacco smoke and pollutants.
- Drugs like aspirin.

} chemical neotoxins

- Stress, emotion, anger and excitement.

} mental neotoxins

How can I identify which neotoxins are trigger factors for my asthma?

There are two ways to do this. First, see which activity, places and times are associated with the asthma attacks. You should fill in an environmental diary (see Chapter 6) and then correlate activity, place and time with asthma attack. An asthma attack may occur immediately after exposure to a neotoxin, but sometimes the response is delayed for up to 24 hours.

Second, by putting a small amount of a specially prepared neotoxin solution, e.g. pollen, onto the skin of your forearm and pricking the skin with a needle. If you are allergic to a substance then a small white lump called a wheal will usually arise around the needle prick. This test is not totally reliable and will only show the presence of extrinsic asthma-type allergy which usually occurs in childhood or early adult life. Approximately 50 per cent of adults and 90 per cent of children with asthma show positive skin tests. Intrinsic asthma does not usually show on skin testing, tends to start at the age of 30 plus, and continues in later life. Extrinsic asthma usually improves considerably when you reduce the total load of neotoxins, whereas intrinsic asthma is less responsive to this approach.

How can I tell if my asthma attack is severe?

This is always a decision that should be made by a doctor. However, if you see any of the following symptoms, call medical help immediately, day or night (asthma is usually much worse at night):

- Inability to speak;
- Sweating;
- Blue lips and pale complexion;
- Drowsiness;
- No better after medication.

Do not postpone medical attention, since most asthma deaths occur due to underestimating the severity of the attack and so delaying in getting adequate treatment.

ALLERGIC RHINITIS

What is Allergic Rhinitis?

Allergic rhinitis is a recurrent condition affecting the nose. The symptoms include:

Sneezing
Blocked nose
Watery
discharge

} Patients will suffer from 2 out of 3 of these symptoms often for more than 1 hour

The eyes are also usually affected, and water and itch. Common trigger factors that start an attack of allergic rhinitis include:

The house dust mite
Animal fur and saliva
Fungi
Pollen (which causes hayfever)
Some foods, e.g. cows' milk.

Sometimes it can be difficult to tell the difference between allergic rhinitis and a cold. Table 7.2 will enable you to distinguish the one from the other.

If you notice the activity, time and place where you suffer most from allergic rhinitis then you will get a good clue as to the origin of the allergy (see Table 7.3). Remember that although allergic rhinitis usually occurs straight after exposure, if the problem is food, there may be a delay of up to 24 hours before symptoms occur.

How can I reduce the risk of suffering allergic rhinitis?

The likelihood of allergic rhinitis can be greatly reduced by removing the source of the allergy. Pollen and hay fever are dealt with in the next section. After the cause has been identified, the following measures can be taken to reduce exposure.

Animals
- Don't allow pets in your bedroom. Let them live, sleep and be groomed in part of the house that you can avoid;
- Keep pets in an area that can be easily washed (e.g. linoleum), since this will prevent build-up of animal hairs;
- Avoid situations and occupations where you will come into contact with animals, e.g. pet owners and their houses, zoos, circuses, farmers and vets;
- Don't buy pets in future.

Feathers
Feathers come from live birds but are also found in pillows, cushions, quilts and eiderdowns, which should all be avoided by people with feather allergy.

House dust mite
House dust mites are microscopic transparent insects ($\frac{1}{3}$ mm long), that produce faecal particles 1 micron in diameter that are able to travel right into the lung. The mites are usually at their highest level in the bedroom and live in mattresses, upholstery, carpets and curtains. They feed on human skin scales, and an adult person loses 1g of scales a day. The average mattress has of the order of 10,000 to 100,000 house dust mites in it. House dust mites prefer warm moist places, which are encouraged by modern construction methods emphasizing small rooms, low ventilation with high insulation, and humidity. House dust mites can be greatly reduced by:

- Living in a house that is dry and sited away from open water and underground streams;
- Avoiding open fires that burn coal, gas and paraffin which produce a lot of water vapour increasing humidity;
- Ensuring good ventilation, especially in the bedroom, to avoid the build up of humidity;
- Buy a new mattress preferably without buttons and have it on a wooden frame rather than a divan;
- Remove feather-filled pillows and eider-downs. Replace them with cellular cotton blankets and sleep on a pillow case stuffed with another cotton blanket;
- If you sleep in a bunk bed, take the upper bed.

The other measures to reduce house dust mites are all down to *housework*, which ideally should

Table 7.2 **Rhinitis and cold symptoms**

Symptoms of allergic rhinitis	Symptoms of a 'cold'
Sudden onset	More gradual onset
Frequent sneezing (often within seconds)	Sneezing rare
Clear watery discharge	Yellow discharge
Eyes also affected	Eyes usually spared

Table 7.3 **Time/Place where allergy is worse, and likely cause**

Time of year/day when allergy is worse	Place where allergy is worse	Cause of allergy
February to May	Outside, especially near fields and woods	Tree pollen
May to July		Grass pollen
July to October		Weed pollen
July and August		Cereals
All year round with peak August to October	Outdoors in *damp* places and near water	Fungal spores
All year round with peak August to October	Indoors in *damp* places, e.g. bathrooms and basements and near water	Fungal spores
All year round seasonal peak in moulting season	Indoors especially near animal's sleeping place	Pet furs and feathers
All year round with peak in winter	Indoors especially in old damp houses, near open water and underground streams	House dust mites
In winter	Indoors	Any form of indoor pollution

be carried out by someone who is not allergic to the house dust mite.

- Vacuum all around the bed and mattress each week. Also vacuum other furniture and in crevices. Use a cylinder vacuum cleaner with a disposable paper dustbag or, even better, a vacuum cleaner with a water filled trap to filter the exhaust air. Upright vacuum cleaners with cloth bags often merely throw the house dust mite into the atmosphere and are counter-productive. Don't forget to vacuum *all* beds in the room. Vacuuming removes the house dust mite but does not remove the sticky eggs, which remain in the mattress.

- Wash all the sheets, blankets, pillow cases and any furry toys taken to bed, once a week. Use a boil wash as the house dust mite eggs are heat resistant.

- Damp dust all surfaces in the room, e.g. window ledges, tops of furniture, pelmets. Don't use a dry brush, since it propels house dust mites into the atmosphere.

- Air your mattress once a month. The house dust mite dislikes sunlight and dry air. If the weather is very cold but dry, then air your mattress outside, since the intense cold kills the house dust mite. House dust mites cannot live in dry, cold conditions and at higher altitudes such as are found in alpine areas.

- Do *not* use insecticides to kill the house dust mite. It is often ineffective and the insecticide may cause you to suffer a chemical sensitivity.

Fungal spores

The way to avoid fungal spores is to avoid wet and damp places at home and work. Fungi release many spores in wet conditions, especially early in the morning in July and August. Spores are also released by grass cutting and other agricultural work. Fungi can be reduced by heat, ventilation and frost. Do *not* use fungicides, since they may cause you to suffer a chemical sensitivity.

HAY FEVER

Pollens and hay fever

About 1 in 5 of the population suffer from hay fever at some time in their life. It is commonest in the teens and usually causes problems in June/July, during exam time. Pollens tend not to cause asthma because they are too large (20–200 microns in diameter) to get into the lungs. However, they do cause allergic symptoms, such as watery eyes and sore throat, within about 2 minutes of contact.

Paradoxically, hay fever is becoming more common, despite the fact that the amount of pollen in the atmosphere is getting less. This is due to the great increase in the level of all the neotoxins. A hay fever sufferer will react to a concentration of 50 pollen grains per cubic metre. During an average summer day there may be 200 pollen grains per cubic metre.

Hay fever may be caused by tree pollens, grass pollens and weed pollens. The tree pollen season lasts roughly from February to May, the grass pollen season lasts from May to July, and the weed pollen season runs from July to October.

The way to reduce your exposure to pollen is to:

- Try to avoid going out on warm sunny days during the hay fever season. The pollen count is highest midmorning and late afternoon/evening;
- Sleep with your bedroom windows closed;
- When you are travelling by car or train, keep the windows closed;
- Stay in the towns and avoid indoor pollinating plants. This is one of the few

occasions when air conditioning may help your health;

- Stay away from fields, and don't cut the grass;
- Wear dark glasses that tend to keep pollen away from your eyes;
- Be aware that rain *during* the pollen season reduces the pollen count. Rain *before* the pollen season increases the pollen count;
- Holiday at the seaside (low pollen count) or at a place where the grass is not in season e.g. June, July in the Southern hemisphere. Hilly and mountainous areas with turbulent air flow, e.g. alpine areas are much better than plains.

What is 'rape seed flu'?

There is a particularly virulent form of hay fever caused by rape, a bright yellow plant grown for oil and animal feed. This plant is actually insect pollinated but is able to produce a severe form of hay fever resembling influenza in people living near fields of it. 'Rape seed flu' is becoming much more common because the area under cultivation has risen dramatically in the past 10 years. The cause of the 'rape seed flu' is usually the aromatic substances that the oil seed rape gives off, and in some cases is also due to poisoning by pesticides and other chemicals applied to the plants throughout the growing cycle.

Are sinusitis and glue ear caused by allergy?

Sinusitis (an inflammation of the sinuses of the face) and glue ear (extra mucous secretion in the middle ear) are commonly caused by food allergy. Sinusitis and glue ear will often improve after removing *all* cows' milk, dairy products and beef from the diet. Removing dairy products from the diet makes the mucous in the sinuses and nose more runny and less likely to accumulate and cause sinusitis and glue ear.

Sinusitis may be encouraged by the presence of nasal polyps which are small soft finger shaped lumps which start to grow within the nose. These polyps cover over the entrance to the sinus and cause sinusitis. Polyp growth occurs due to chronic exposure to the house dust mite, fungi or similar allergic substance.

SKIN CONDITIONS

The skin is the largest organ in the body and covers 1.5 square metres in adults in adults. There are four common allergic skin conditions:

Atopic eczema
Psoriasis
Contact dermatitis
Urticaria or hives

Atopic eczema

Atopic eczema affects at least 1 person in 20 at some time in their lives. Eczema causes scaly cracks in the flexures, e.g. elbows and knee joints. An atopic person is one likely to react to common substances in an allergic way, e.g. asthma, eczema, hay fever. Half of all child eczema sufferers are atopic.

Is eczema inherited or due to acquired factors?

Although eczema is partly inherited, it is also related to the mother's diet during pregnancy and the child's diet after birth. Mothers who either avoid eating a monotonous repetitive diet or else reduce, or even completely avoid allergic foods, (such as cows' milk and dairy products, eggs, fish, peanuts, soya beans, citrus fruit, chocolate, tomatoes and nuts), are much less likely to have children with eczema. Breast fed children are less likely to have eczema, especially if the mother has a low allergy diet. Bottle fed children who are given cows' milk are considerably more likely to have eczema than breast fed children. The bottle feed that is least likely to cause eczema is called caesin hydrolysate (i.e. milk that has already been partly digested).

Is eczema becoming more common?

Eczema is a disease of twentieth-century western civilization. In England it is now six times more common than it was during the Second World War. The main reason for this dramatic increase in eczema has been the large rise in the level of neotoxins, especially food additives.

How should I treat my eczema?

If you are a pregnant mother, you can lower the likelihood of your child getting eczema by reducing and rotating highly allergic foods in your diet and breast feeding your child. If you are an adult, try the exclusion diet on page 172, with the supplements that are recommended.

Psoriasis

This is a common skin condition affecting 1 in 50 people, often inherited. It causes a red, scaly rash that particularly affects the outside of knees and elbows, and the scalp. There are several trigger factors which may precipitate an attack of psoriasis:

- Infections, especially a sore throat and local fungal infections of the skin (biological neotoxin);
- Drugs, e.g. antibiotics tablets, beta-blockers for raised blood pressure and lithium (chemical neotoxin);
- Stress, e.g. an accident or injury, other illness, climatic changes or hormonal changes (mental neotoxins).

How should I treat my psoriasis?

Avoid as many trigger factors listed above as possible. Try the exclusion diet listed on page 172. Also take the supplements advised.

Contact dermatitis

This is an allergic skin condition that is usually related to *direct contact* to a neotoxin. Contact dermatitis accounts for 40 per cent of all occupational illness, and usually takes a minimum of 12 to 48 hours to develop. Contact dermatitis may be caused by two different processes, chemical and physical irritation, and allergy. It is often difficult to distinguish between these two processes. Contact dermatitis is not linked to atopy; however, the rash is very similar to atopic eczema. The factor that helps you to guess the cause of the contact dermatitis is its distribution.

Common agents causing irritant contact dermatitis include water; metals, especially nickel; acids and alkalis, soaps and detergents; petrochemicals, solvents, paints and glues; polishes and cleaners, food acids, and physical factors such as heat, cold and ultra-violet light. Common agents causing allergic contact dermatitis include foods and plants; feathers and woods; drugs; rubber chemicals; plastics, leathers, cement; adhesives, glues and varnishes; cosmetics, creams and lotions.

The table opposite lists the distribution of contact dermatitis with its most likely cause. Chemical irritant contact dermatitis usually affects hands, where allergic contact dermatitis usually affects face, necks and eyelids.

It is possible to test for allergic contact dermatitis by patch testing. Possible allergic substances are taped to the back for 2 days. The back is examined after a further 2 days and allergic substances will produce a reaction. Patch testing involves a different and slower allergic mechanism than prick testing.

Table 7.4 **Contact dermatitis**

Site of the body affected	Likely cause of contact dermatitis
Scalp	Hair applications, e.g. shampoos, hair dyes and bleaches
Face	Women — cosmetics } and Men — aftershaves } soaps Also spectacles may cause rash on face
Eyelids	Cosmetics, hair sprays, and hand allergens (due to rubbing eyes)
Lips	Lipsticks, toothpaste and mouthwash
Ears	Earrings, especially nickel, clothes, detergents and aftershaves
Armpit	Deodorants, hair removers, clothes, soaps and detergents
Hands (two thirds of all contact dermatitis affects hands, especially webs of fingers)	Occupational chemicals, soaps and detergents, rubber gloves, lotions and creams
Body	Soaps and detergents, clothes, leather, rubber, nickel especially bra clips, watches, jean studs
Genital (women)	Medications and contraceptives (all sorts), deodorants and applications, pads and tampons
Genital (men)	Medications and contraceptives (all sorts)
Feet	Footwear, rubber, medications

How do I cure contact dermatitis?

There are two stages to curing contact dermatitis:

- **Identification:** find the substance that causes the contact dermatitis by noting distribution of rash, and correlate it with chemicals touching that area.
- **Avoidance:** avoid contact with the allergic substance. Do this either by removing it from your environment, e.g changing cosmetics, or else by using proper protective precautions, e.g. gloves, barrier creams or better ventilation.

Urticaria

Urticaria, or 'hives', is a rapidly occurring (usually within minutes), allergic reaction that occurs in small blood vessels in the skin. It gives rise to:

- a 'nettle rash' (white raised lumps in the skin);
- itching and burning.

Urticaria can be caused by every class of neotoxin which can either be eaten or inhaled, or else come into direct contact with the skin. The common culprits include:

- **Biological neotoxins**
  Seafoods (especially shellfish and bony fish, e.g. cod and mackerel), berries (especially strawberries), chocolate and cocoa, nuts, (especially peanuts, cashews and hazelnuts), pulses, eggs, citrus fruits, dairy products (especially cheese), cereals (white sugar and flour), tomatoes, potatoes, onions, preserved meat, chinese food, spices, fresh apples, bananas, cherries, grapes, mangos, melons, pineapple, rhubarb and raisin, yeast and yeast products (e.g. bovril, marmite, oxo, vegemite), cold and alcoholic drinks, tinned and packed foods, all food additives, especially azo dyes.

  Infections (bacterial, viral, fungal and parasites).

  Animals (fur, flesh and feathers), insects (especially bees, wasps and house dust mites), pollens.
- **Chemical neotoxins**
  Formaldehyde, drugs (especially salicylates and antibiotics), vitamins, toothpaste, cosmetics, toiletries, hair preparations and aerosols, tobacco smoke, sulphur dioxide.
- **Physical neotoxins**
  Heat, cold and ultra violet light
- **Mental neotoxins**
  Stress, emotion, excitement and anger

Why does urticaria occur?

Urticaria occurs due to the release of *histamine* and other vasoactive amines (i.e. substances that cause small blood vessels to dilate). The histamine is either released by the neotoxin or else, as in the case of several foods, the histamine or the vasoactive amine is already present in the food.

How should I treat my urticaria?

Urticaria is a variable disease. It may come suddenly and disappear equally suddenly. The way to beat urticaria is first, to keep an environmental diary (see page 142). Then, at the first appearance of a nettle rash, look back up to 24 hours to try and identify the culprit. As a last resort, an antihistamine will usually control urticaria, but in the long-term the cure is to remove the offending agent.

THE SUPERHEALTH EXCLUSION DIET FOR ASTHMA, ECZEMA AND PSORIASIS

Completely exclude for 2 weeks the following:

All dairy products, including cheese
Eggs
Beef, pork and lamb
Fish
Wheat and wheat products
Bread and all cereal products
Oats, barley and rye
Tomatoes
Onions
Citrus fruits
Pineapple
Bananas
Nuts
Chocolate and cocoa
Sugar and salt
Yeast, vinegar and sauces
Coffee
Tea
All colourings, flavourings and preservatives (All E numbers)
All soft drinks
All alcoholic drinks
Tap water

It is very important to try and give up smoking.

NB. This is *not* a permanent diet, but an exclusion diet for a 2 week trial.

Supplements to be taken are as follows: (For adults)

Vitamin A	5,000 iu	daily
Vitamin B_1	50 mg	daily
Vitamin B_2	50 mg	daily
Vitamin B_3	100 mg	daily
Vitamin B_5	100 mg	daily
Vitamin B_6	50 mg	daily
Vitamin B_{12}	1,000 mcg	by injection *weekly* for 4 weeks
Vitamin C	2,000 mg	(during asthmatic attack 4,000 to 8,000 mg) daily

Vitamin E	200 iu	daily
Magnesium	500 mg	daily
Zinc	15 mg	daily
Cod Liver Oil	10 ml	daily
Evening Primrose	1,500 mg	daily

Drink at least 3–4 pints of pure spring water a day.

Caution: These vitamin and mineral supplements should only be taken by patients who have received clearance from their own doctor.

CHAPTER EIGHT

BEATING ARTHRITIS AND RHEUMATISM

ARTHRITIS AND RHEUMATISM

Arthritis is a very broad term that does not specify cause, but just means any pain in a joint. Rheumatism is an even broader term and means any pain in a bone, joint, muscle, ligament, tendon or cartilage. These structures, in spite of their completely different appearances, are all made of the same substance called connective tissue. Arthritis is very common, and affects about one in seven adults in the western world.

The basic disease process in arthritis is *inflammation* of a joint, which becomes:

red
swollen
hot
tender, and
painful.

In rheumatism, the other connective tissue structures become similarly inflamed. The disease process in arthritis and rheumatism is also very complex; it includes the release of

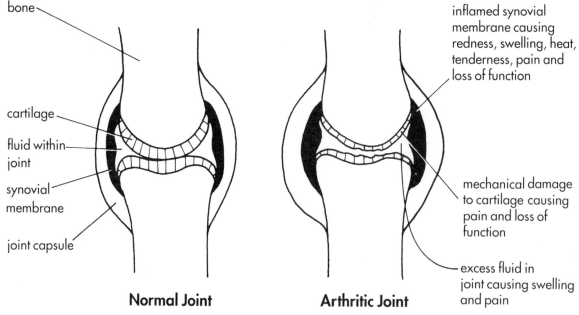

Figure 8.1 **Joint changes in arthritis**

free radicals, and also damaging local hormones called prostaglandins and kinins. Figure 8.1 illustrates the structure of a normal joint, and one with arthritis.

There are three different ways in which arthritis may occur: to an extent these causes overlap.

- **Mechanical damage to a joint surface**
  An accident at any time in life that damages a joint surface encourages the development of arthritis. Mechanical damage may also occur slowly if a joint is overloaded (e.g. through being overweight) or overused (e.g. dancers' joints), or not being optimally used (e.g. a congenital problem or fracture that leaves one leg much shorter than the other).
- **Biochemical abnormalities**
  These can be divided into those that occur due to a recognized disease (usually an enzyme deficiency, e.g. gout, where the body is unable to process a usually occurring substance). Then there are those due to neo-toxins, e.g. allergic foods and the joint is affected.
- **Autoimmune and other joint diseases**
  Rheumatoid arthritis, which is mostly an autoimmune disease, tends to be much more common in women than in men. It occurs because the body produces antibodies to its own joints. These autoimmune antibodies damage joints and cause pain and limitation in movement. Autoimmune arthritis can be triggered and made worse by neotoxins.

The effects of these three sources of arthritis are additive. The overall likelihood of suffering from arthritis is the sum of the three sources as shown in Figure 8.2.

A moderate amount of mechanical damage to a joint, or a similar amount of biochemical abnormality are, on their own, not enough to cause arthritis. However, when taken together they are enough to pass the threshold, and consequently arthritis occurs.

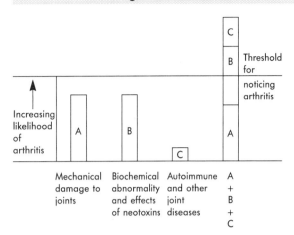

Figure 8.2 **Likelihood of arthritis**

What is the importance of fats and oils causing or curing arthritis?

The fats you eat are a very important factor in deciding whether or not you will suffer from arthritis. One simple explanation of arthritis is that there is a lack of the right lubricating oils within the joint and that causes the pain. Consequently, you can help your arthritis by increasing your oil intake but you must make sure that it is the right sort of oil. The types that help arthritis are the Essential Fatty Acids (EFA), which only occur in the unsaturated form. The ones that tend to make arthritis worse are the saturated and unsaturated non-essential fatty acids see Figure 8.3.

The Omega-3 essential fatty acids can be obtained from oily fish like sardines, mackerel, tuna, salmon, herring and trout. It is also present in linseed oil, provided that it has been cold-pressed.

Omega-6 essential fatty acids are present in evening primrose oil, sunflower and sunflower oil (not margarine), and sesame and almond oil. It is important to have your oils cold-pressed, as the usual extraction process and frying denature the oils and make them much less useful.

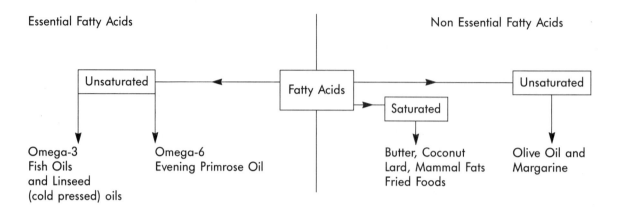

Essential Fatty Acids | Non Essential Fatty Acids

Unsatured ← Fatty Acids → Saturated → Unsaturated

Omega-3 Fish Oils and Linseed (cold pressed) oils

Omega-6 Evening Primrose Oil

Butter, Coconut Lard, Mammal Fats Fried Foods

Olive Oil and Margarine

Can chemicals cause arthritis?

Chemicals such as central heating fumes, motor vehicle exhaust fumes and the chlorine in tap water can frequently cause or exacerbate arthritis. If you have not improved with the following arthritis exclusion diet (see below) then you will have to test yourself for chemical sensitivity (see Chapter 3).

The Superhealth treatment for arthritis and rheumatism is similar whether the underlying cause is mechanical, biochemical, auto-immune or a mixed cause. It consists of:

- Reducing the total load of neotoxins by having clean air, clean food and clean water;
- Particularly reducing the neotoxin(s) to which you are especially susceptible. These are mostly foods and they can be avoided by going onto an exclusion diet for 2 weeks. This exclusion diet initially involves removing a large number of foods in order to identify the culprit(s). However, over 75 per cent of those people with arthritis may gain relief from pain by suitable food exclusion;
- Using sleep and rest, exercise, vitamin, mineral and other supplements to return to health. Regular gentle stretching exercises are an important part of restoring full mobility to any joint. Essential fatty acids, especially fish oils, are invaluable in producing pain free function to arthritic joints.

It may take over 4 weeks for a joint completely to empty itself of accumulated neotoxins. Consequently, joint pain takes a long time to disappear. Similarly, during the challenge stage, because it takes such a long time for neotoxins in the blood to get into the joint, there may be a long delay, up to 48 hours, before an arthritis returns after a food challenge.

Arthritis Exclusion Diet

Completely exclude the following:

All flour (brown and white)
All flour products
All western grains (barley, corns, oats and rye)
White sugar and all yeast products
All mammal meat (beef, lamb, pork – all forms)
Milk and milk products
Cheese
Eggs
Chocolate and cocoa

Citrus fruits
Apple and pear skin, berries
Tomatoes, potatoes and all peppers
Onions
All lentils and beans including soya
Vinegar
Pepper
Herbs and spices
Coffee
Tea
Salt, sugar and artificial sweetener
Alcoholic drinks
Soft drinks
All tinned and frozen food
All additives (E numbers)
Tap water

It is important to give up smoking.

Supplements to be taken are as follows: (for adults)

Vitamin B_1	50 mg	daily
Vitamin B_2	50 mg	daily
Vitamin B_3	100 mg	daily
Vitamin B_5	100 mg	daily
Vitamin B_6	50 mg	daily
Vitamin C	2,000 mg	daily
Vitamin E	200 iu	daily
Calcium	500 mg	daily
Magnesium	250 mg	daily
Cod Liver Oil	10 ml	twice
(Omega-3 oils)		a day
Evening Primrose	2,000 mg	daily
(Omega-6 oils)		

Drink 3 to 4 pints of spring water (not fizzy) every day.

Caution: These vitamin and mineral supplements should only be taken by patients who have received clearance from their own doctor.

CHAPTER NINE

BEATING COLITIS AND BOWEL PROBLEMS

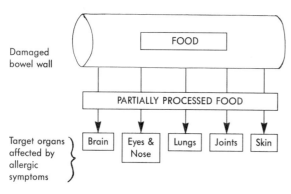

Figure 9.1 **Allergic symptoms caused by bowel problems**

THE BOWEL AND ALLERGIC SYMPTOMS IN MAJOR ORGANS

Food allergy may affect all the major organs of the body. However, almost all food allergies start because of problems with either diet and/or the bowel. In either case the bowel is unable to process fully all the food eaten. An allergy starts after the malfunctioning bowel wall lets unprocessed food into the blood stream, where it induces a reaction in the immune and detoxification systems which itself may be defective. If the diet is more suitable and the bowel is able to completely process foods *before* they enter the body, then the likelihood of allergy drops dramatically.

The bowel wall can become damaged by both inherited and acquired factors.

Inherited factors
An inherited enzyme defect such as 'lactase deficiency' which stops the bowel from digesting cows milk sugar (lactose).

Acquired factors
- **Biological neotoxins**
  Repetitive over-exposure to food, e.g. milk, wheat.
  Infections of the bowel, especially viral, bacterial, and enteritis.
  Fungal infections such as candida (see Chapter 10).
- **Chemical neotoxins**
  Massive chemical over-exposure after a chemical spill.
  Repeated use of antibiotics.
- **Physical neotoxins**
  Massive radiation overdose, usually causes death for other reasons.
- **Mental neotoxins**
  Stress, accident, surgery, pregnancy.

The immune system also may be defective, especially in the first 6 months of life. Breast-feeding helps an infant over this period, since mother's milk contains many helpful antibodies. Bottle fed babies have a much higher incidence of allergies.

Which bowel diseases are allergic?

The alimentary canal from mouth to anus can be thought of as one very long organ. Allergy can affect any part independently, or several parts simultaneously. For example, aphthous mouth ulcers and teething are often associated with diarrhoea and irritation around the anus.

Bowel diseases caused by allergy include:

Aphthous mouth ulcers
Indigestion
Crohn's disease
Ulcerative colitis
Irritable bowel
Coeliac disease
Haemorrhoids or piles

How can I treat my Irritable Bowel?

Almost half of all patients attending gastroenterology (bowel) clinics are given a diagnosis of 'irritable bowel', and about two thirds of these patients are women.

The common symptoms of 'irritable bowel' include:

- Colic (abdominal pain), reduced by opening bowels or passing wind;
- Abdominal distension and flatulence;
- Diarrhoea especially before or after breakfast;
- Constipation; this may alternate with diarrhoea.

The symptoms of irritable bowel are made worse by stress and the wrong diet.

Approximately two thirds of irritable bowel patients will improve on the correct exclusion diet. An exclusion diet is given at the end of this chapter which can be used in conjunction with the Superhealth plan. If irritable bowel is not treated, it may progress to other more serious bowel diseases.

Will Crohn's disease improve on an exclusion diet?

Over half of patients with Crohn's disease will improve if the offending food substance is removed from their diet. Despite permanent damage to their bowel, these patients can gain a dramatic improvement in health by using the correct exclusion diet.

What is coeliac disease?

This is an inherited disease occurring in both children and adults in which the bowel is unable to process the protein *gluten*, found in wheat and rye, and to a lesser extent in barley and oats.

If a coeliac sufferer eats wheat, the surface of the small bowel is damaged, its area reduced and, consequently, the absorption of other food substances is incomplete. This often produces diarrhoea, weight loss, and in children, failure to grow and develop. Sometimes a tendency to coeliac disease is not revealed until a trigger factor like an accident, infection, surgery or pregnancy occurs. Coeliac disease can be complicated by a skin condition called dermatitis herpetiformis.

Coeliac disease can be controlled by completely avoiding foods containing gluten. This means avoiding all wheat, rye, barley and oats (see page 51), or else eating specially prepared wheat products that have had the gluten removed.

Exclusion diet for bowel conditions

Completely exclude the following:

Milk and all milk products and cheese
All wheat flour and wheat flour products (brown and white)
All other western grains (barley, corn, oats, rye)
Sugar (all forms) and yeast

All mammal meat (beef, lamb, pork – all
    forms)
Eggs
Chocolate and cocoa
Apple and pear skin
Tomatoes
Onions
Lentils (beans, peas, senna and soya beans)
Nuts
Coffee
Tea
Alcohol
Soft drinks
Citrus fruit juices
All tinned and frozen food
All additives
Tap water (for drinking *and* cooking)

Supplements to be taken are as follows: (for adults)

Vitamin A	10,000	iu	daily
Vitamin B$_1$	50	mg	daily
Vitamin B$_2$	50	mg	daily
Vitamin B$_3$	100	mg	daily
Vitamin B$_5$	100	mg	daily
Vitamin B$_6$	50	mg	daily
Vitamin B$_{12}$	1,000	mcg	monthly
Vitamin C	3,000	mg	daily
Vitamin D	400	iu	daily
Vitamin E	200	iu	daily
Folic Acid	0.4	mg	daily
Calcium	500	mg	daily
Magnesium	500	mg	daily
Zinc	30	mg	daily
Acidophilus	3	tabs	daily

Drink 3 to 4 pints of bottled spring water a day.

Caution: These vitamins and mineral supplements should only be taken by patients who have received clearance from their own doctor.

CHAPTER TEN

BEATING RECURRENT TIREDNESS, ME AND CANDIDA ALBICANS

CANDIDA ALBICANS

Ecological balance is a fundamentally import-ant concept in nature. This balance exists at many levels, from the individual cell to the whole planet earth, which some scientists suggest acts like a self-regulating living being (the Gaia concept).

Each human body and each organ system has a similar level of self-regulating balance. For example, the normal large bowel is not sterile but has balanced numbers of bacteria and candida albicans (yeasts). Symptoms and diseases arise when this delicate balance is disturbed. The way that we live in the twentieth century tips the scales strongly in favour of candida.

Excess candida in the bowel has a toxic effect on the immune and detoxification systems. This is due to the release of poisonous chemicals, including aldehyde, which are produced by the candida and released into the bowel. These chemicals are then absorbed into the bloodstream and act on the brain and other target organs to produce allergies. The more yeast present in the bowel, the greater the challenge to the immune and detoxification systems. Even a normal immune and detoxification system cannot withstand the load of neotoxins arising from a chronic candida infection.

If the body is simultaneously assaulted by other neotoxins, then the immune and detoxification systems are unable to do their usual thorough jobs, and allow many more allergic substances to remain in the blood-

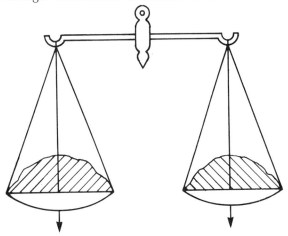

Bacteria especially Lactobacillus increased by good health, organic diet, live yoghurt, vitamins and minerals, exercise

Fungi especially Candida increased by poor health, yeast-containing foods, sugar and sweet foods, wheat and carbohydrates, antibiotics, steroids, oral contraceptives, multiple pregnancies, diabetes, fungi at work and home

Figure 10.1 **Bacteria/fungal ecological balance in the bowel**

stream. These cause allergies in target organs distant from the bowel, e.g., brain, lungs, skin.

Candida also encourages allergies because it causes mechanical damage to the bowel wall, allowing undigested food and fungal poisons to enter the bloodstream and further compromise the immune system.

What disease and symptoms can be caused by candida albicans?

Candida albicans is able to produce all the classic allergic disease symptoms (see page 20). Some of the commoner hallmarks of chronic candida infection are:

- Recurrent tiredness often seems to occur due to the toxic effect of a high load of candida. It is similar to the ME symptom;
- Many mental symptoms, including headache, poor memory and concentration, confusion, irritability, mood swings, depression;
- Addictions including alcoholism, craving for sugary or starchy foods;
- Bowel problems including abdominal pain and distension, diarrhoea and constipation;
- Aching muscles and joints;
- Frequent fungal infections especially of genitals, mouth and skin (e.g. thrush);
- Pre-menstrual tension.

Which factors make a candida infection more likely?

Genetic susceptibility

Some people are more vulnerable to candida due to an inherited enzyme defect.

General state of health, including state of immune and detoxification systems

Good health is promoted by eating an organic diet and taking adequate amounts of exercise and vitamin and mineral supplements. The general state of health is related to total load of neotoxins and individual neotoxins to which the body is especially susceptible.

Amount of yeast contained in the food in the diet

Many foods contain yeast. A full list is given opposite. The common sources include beer and wine, vinegar, yeast extracts, mushrooms and cheeses.

Foods encouraging the growth of yeast

These include all foods containing a high proportion of sugar or refined (white) flour. Candida needs sugar to grow, however, providing that there are adequate supplies it is able potentially to increase its weight 100 times in 24 hours.

Antibiotics

These may be given as medication or may be a contaminant, especially of meats. Antibiotics are made from fungi and, consequently, kill bacteria but do not harm fungi. Broad spectrum antibiotics, such as ampicillin, amoxicillin and tetracyclines are the worst, especially when they are not fully absorbed into the body but remain within the bowel. A course of more than 2 months or more than 4 courses in a year are likely to induce a chronic candida infection of the bowel.

Steroids

Steroids e.g. hydrocortisone (as tablets *or* cream), prednisone and prednisolone, if taken long term, all suppress the immune and detoxification systems and reduce the ability to fight candida.

The oral contraceptive

The oral contraceptive contains sex steroids and, consequently has many effects on the body. It tends to suppress the immune and detoxification systems, and makes sugar more easily available to the candida, encouraging multiplication of numbers. Taking the oral contraceptive for more than about 1 year encourages chronic candida infections.

Multiple pregnancies

Pregnancy causes a massive rise in the level of sex hormones, which greatly encourages growth of candida.

Diabetes

Diabetics have a raised blood sugar which greatly encourages the growth of candida.

How can I stop suffering from candida albicans?

This can be a long process, however, the following measures are helpful:

- Follow the Superhealth plan and reduce your total load of neotoxins by getting clean food, clean air and clean water.
- Also remove the neotoxins to which you are particularly susceptible. Then use exercise with vitamin and mineral supplements to get yourself back to full health.
- Avoid all yeast containing foods, (see list below). Instead, eat foods like 'live' yoghurt which contain lactobacillus. This is a bacteria that normally lives in the gut and competes with candida for nutrients, keeping the level of candida low. This bacteria is found naturally in 'live' yogurt but can be taken in tablet or powder form when it is called acidophilus.
- Avoid all sugary foods and foods containing a high proportion of unrefined (white) starch or flour, (see list on page 51).
- Take vitamins and other supplements. Vitamin B, Biotin and Folic Acid keep the candida in a less invasive (non-mycelial) form. The immune and detoxification systems are given a boost by vitamins A, C

and E; and trace metals, zinc and copp Make sure all vitamins are yeast free. Many vitamins, especially Vitamin B are often made from yeast.

- Don't take broad spectrum antibiotics unless absolutely necessary. Eat organic food, especially organic meat, which does not contain antibiotics.
- Don't take steroids unless absolutely necessary.
- Try to use some method of contraception other than the oral contraceptive. Failing that try not to take the oral contraceptive continuously for more than 6 months at a time without a 3 month break.
- Avoid fungi in your home and work. Fungi do not like airing and ventilation, dryness, heat, and sunlight. Fungi grow best in wet, dark, poorly ventilated places such as bathrooms and showers, under sinks, damp cupboards, damp beds, refrigerators, cellars and basements, gardens and compost heaps.

CANDIDA-FREE DIET

The key sources of candida are alcohol, vinegar, meat and cheese. Avoid the following completely:

- Alcoholic drinks (all types, including 'low alcohol')
- Antibiotics and products containing antibiotics, i.e. non-organic meat.
- Bread (all bread and bread products except soda bread)
- Buns and cakes and mince pies
- Cheese (all forms), cottage cheese, cream cheese, sour cream, sour milk, yoghurt, buttermilk
- Chocolate
- Coffee
- Cream crackers, Twiglets (contain cheese)
- Fish – smoked or pickled

over →

- Fruit – dried and overripe
- Fruit juice (bottled, canned, frozen or packaged) – fresh home squeezed citrus juices are candida free
- Grapes, currants, sultanas, raisins, plums, dates, prunes and all products containing these.
- Malted drinks – Ovaltine, Horlicks
- Meat products containing bread – beefburgers, meat loaf, sausages, smoked or pickled meat
- Melon
- Monosodium glutamate and Chinese food
- Mushrooms and truffles
- Pies
- Pizzas
- *Raw* root vegetables (that grow *under* the soil), beets, carrots, onion, potatoes, turnips
- Soups (tinned and packet)
- Tea
- Vinegar and vinegar containing foods, i.e. pickled foods, sauces, relishes, ketchups, salad dressings, mayonnaise, horseradish
- Vitamins and any vitamin fortified food – most B vitamins are made from yeast unless otherwise stated
- Yeast extracts – Bovril, gravy browning, marmite, stock cubes, vegemite

Suggested vitamin and mineral supplements for Candida problems in adults

Vitamin A	10,000	iu	daily
Vitamin B_1	50	mg	daily
Vitamin B_2	50	mg	daily
Vitamin B_3	100	mg	daily
Vitamin B_5	100	mg	daily
Vitamin B_6	50	mg	daily
Vitamin B_{12}	1,000	mcg	monthly
Folic Acid	0.4	mg	daily
Biotin	500	mcg	daily
Vitamin C	3,000	mg	daily
Vitamin E	200	iu	daily
Magnesium	500	mg	daily
Iron	200	mg	daily
Zinc	30	mg	daily
Evening Primrose Oil	1,500	mg	daily
Acidophilus	4 tablets		daily
Potassium (Elemental)	100	mg	daily

Drink 3 to 4 pints of bottled spring water a day.

Caution: These vitamin and mineral supplements should only be taken by patients who have received clearance from their own doctor.

How can I beat vaginal thrush?

As well as the general measures suggested in the previous section, there are several specific local measures that can reduce the risk of vaginal thrush:

- Wear skirts, stockings and cotton underwear. Candida likes to grow in warm, moist areas. Wearing nylon underwear or trousers or tights reduces ventilation and encourages thrush.
- Avoid broken skin. Candida is able to invade if skin or mucus membrane is broken after scratching. Avoid everything that could cause irritation, e.g. bubble bath, perfumes, soaps, vaginal deodorants, irritant contraceptives, applicators and gels.
- Always wash and wipe from front to back. This avoids contaminating the vulva with candida from the anal passage.
- Before sex use plenty of lubrication to prevent broken vaginal mucous membranes. After sex wash away semen by using a vaginal douche. Growth of candida is encouraged by semen.

IS MYALGIC ENCEPHALOMYELITIS (ME) AN ALLERGIC CONDITION?

ME, otherwise known as 'Yuppie flu' is nature's way of letting us know that the modern urban lifestyle is fundamentally flawed. The typical ME sufferer is a young woman, in her late teens to early forties, who suffers from recurrent tiredness, especially after exercise.

Although viral infections have been suggested as the sole cause of ME, the diverse symptom picture strongly suggests an 'allergic' problem. In ME, in common with allergies, the immune and detoxification systems are not working properly, and the symptoms are often greatly relieved by reducing the total load of neotoxins.

All cases of recurrent tiredness should be assessed by a qualified practitioner who, at an early stage, can rule out other important causes, including diabetes, myxoedema, infections (including TB), kidney failure, liver failure, arthritis, depression, side-effects of drugs, anaemia and cancer.

The common symptoms of ME include:

- An initial (prodromal) illness consisting of a flu-like illness affecting the lungs, or bowel and/or other parts. This is then followed by;
- Fatigue and muscular pain especially after exercise. It can often take several days to recover from a bout of exercise;
- Joint pains;
- Recurrent swelling of lymph glands;
- Brain problems including difficulty in concentration, memory, vision and learning, with emotional debility and headaches;
- Bowel problems resembling irritable bowel syndrome with nausea, flatulence and diarrhoea;

- Heart problems including chest pain, palpitations and sweating.

The treatment of ME includes the Superhealth plan, together with *gentle* exercise. It is important to reduce the load of candida and to take vitamin and mineral supplements. Candida, however, is often a symptom rather than a cause of the problem.

Some ME sufferers have symptoms caused by the toxic effects of mercury amalgam in their dental fillings. This mercury poisoning can be helped by removing amalgam fillings and using homoeopathic mercury to aid excretion of stored mercury from the body.

In some cases of ME it is possible to achieve a dramatic improvement in the level of health after the above treatment.

SICK BUILDING SYNDROME

The 'Sick Building Syndrome' is a misnomer, since it is the people who get ill. However, their illness is caused by the building their work in. It is commonest in large, modern, carpeted open-plan offices and shops with sealed windows, air conditioning, fluorescent lights and lots of electronic equipment.

The cause of the illness varies slightly from building to building and, consequently, the symptoms also vary slightly, but include:

Itching or blocked nose
Dry/watery or itchy eyes
Dry throat
Headache
Lethargy

The illness can even progress to:

A 'flu like' illness
Breathlessness
Wheezing

The symptoms are strongly related to the amount of time spent in the building. The

185

symptoms come on after being in the building for several hours and are most noticeable in the afternoon. Symptoms improve after leaving the building and may disappear completely at weekends and during holidays.

Sick building syndrome is caused by neotoxins, many of which are picked up and sprayed onto the occupants by the air conditioning and humidification system. The latter may act as a breeding ground and concentrating mechanism for many neotoxins including:

- **Biological neotoxins**
  Bacterial infections (e.g. Legionnaires disease)
  Viral infections from other occupants
  Fungal, e.g. Aspergillus
  Algal and protozoal – 'causing 'humidifier fever'
  } caused by air conditioning and humidifying systems spraying occupants of building with infection

  Pollen from indoor plants
  House dust mites from carpets
- **Chemical neotoxins**
  Smoking – in open-plan offices
  Formaldehyde from carpets and plasters
  Glues and solvents

Pesticides added to water in air conditioner
- **Physical neotoxins**
  Static electricity caused by dry atmosphere and many plastics
  Radiation from all electric devices
  Fluorescent light (narrow spectrum and flickers)
  Extra low frequency sound waves due to vibration of the building at resonant frequency
- **Mental neotoxin**
  Stress from high pressure job.

The best treatment of sick building syndrome is to change your place of employment. Failing that, follow the Superhealth plan and try to alter as many of the factors as you can to improve your health.

REACTIVE HYPOGLYCAEMIA

There is a particular form of recurrent tiredness called hypoglycaemia (low blood sugar). The low blood sugar periodically occurs due to an excessive amount of sugar and white flour in the diet.

The mechanism by which hypoglycaemia occurs is as follows. A sufferer eats a large

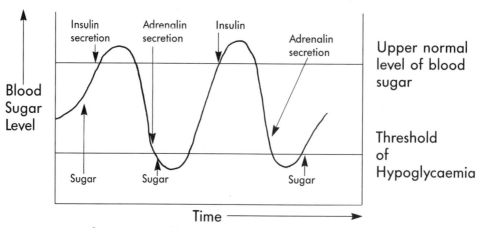

Figure 10.2 **Reactive Hypoglycaemia**

amount of sugar or starchy food; the starch is easily broken into sugar. These sugars are rapidly absorbed from the bowel into the blood and cause the blood glucose level to climb very steeply, above the upper level of blood sugar (Figure 10.2). This raised blood sugar stimulates the pancreas to produce a large amount of the hormone, insulin. The insulin rapidly reduces the blood sugar level by enabling the blood sugar to enter cells all around the body and in this way the high blood sugar level drops. In the absence of insulin, blood sugar cannot enter the cells.

However, the insulin is a long-acting hormone and continues to work even when the blood sugar has been reduced to normal values. Since the initial level of blood sugar was so high, a large amount of insulin has been produced. Consequently, the blood sugar continues to fall and is reduced to a lower than normal level (reactive hypoglycaemia). The low blood sugar then causes a secondary release of the stress hormone adrenalin.

The adrenalin causes a further drop in the already low blood sugar and this induces ravenous hunger and many hypoglycaemia sufferers take more sugar or starch. If a similar high load of sugar is taken again, the blood sugar level will seesaw between high and very low levels, with secretion of adrenalin at each hypoglycaemic episode. After a relatively few cycles of high and low blood sugar, there is no more adrenalin left in the adrenal stores, and the body can no longer be 'pepped', resulting in consequent feelings of weakness.

Other stimulants such as tea, coffee and chocolate can cause release of adrenalin and although, like adrenalin, they initially give a 'lift' in the short term, in the long term they make reactive hypoglycaemia much worse.

Symptoms of hypoglycaemia are very varied but the mains ones include:

- Sweating, especially of the face and palms of hand
- Pallor and tingling especially around the lips
- Palpitations and anxiety
- Tremors

⎫
⎬ Due to the effect of adrenalin
⎭

- Sensations of ravenous hunger
- Recurrent tiredness, weakness, fatigue, sleeplessness, depression
- Appearing drunk (alcohol also induces hypoglycaemia) with poor co-ordination, dizziness, blurring of vision, incoherent speech
- Irritability, mood swings, personality changes, emotional lability, mania, temper outbursts, restlessness
- Headaches
- Poor concentration and memory.

Reactive hypoglycaemia is able to make the following diseases worse:

Alcoholism ⎫
Addictions ⎭ See Chapter 13

Diabetes
Having many reactive hypoglycaemia attacks puts a greater strain on the pancreas, which may eventually fail, causing diabetes.

Migraine
Reactive hypoglycaemia causes dilation of brain blood vessels in an attempt to increase the amount of glucose reaching the brain. Dilated blood vessels cause migraine.

Asthma
Asthma attacks are worse very early in the morning when reactive hypoglycaemia is most likely to occur. Diabetics with high blood sugar are less liable to asthma.

Epilepsy
Fits are common in people with pre-existing epilepsy following hypoglycaemia and alcohol

intake (which induces hypoglycaemia).

Mental illness

Some workers have suggested that hypoglycaemia could be the cause of mental illness, as an inadequate supply of glucose stops the brain from working properly and encourages mental illness. High carbohydrate intake consumes B vitamins, and some patients with mental illness are, in fact, suffering from vitamin deficiency diseases which may be helped by removing high levels of carbohydrates and giving vitamins.

Many food allergies

Many food allergies may be caused through the reduction in general health.

How is Reactive Hypoglycaemia diagnosed?

By taking a *6 hour* glucose tolerance test. This is done by giving a 50g (2 oz) dose of glucose and measuring the blood sugar every hour for 6 hours. The usual 2 hour glucose tolerance test finishes far too soon to show reactive hypoglycaemia.

How can I cure Reactive Hypoglycaemia?

By changing your diet so that you:

- Reduce your total carbohydrate intake. Avoid sugar, chocolate, wheat flour as much as possible;
- Eat 5 or 6 *small* meals per day;
- Eat more protein and fat to make up for lost calories. Many health problems are caused or made worse by excess sugar and starch (carbohydrates) in the diet;
- Make sure that you eat breakfast;
- Avoid alcohol, tobacco, tea, coffee and cocoa, which tend to release adrenalin.

CHAPTER ELEVEN

BEATING MIGRAINE AND NERVOUS SYSTEM DISORDERS

The brain is one of the main target organs for environmental illness. This chapter deals with the physical effects of neotoxins on the brain, Chapter 12 deals with the psychological effects.

MIGRAINE

About 1 woman in 5 and 1 man in 10 suffers from migraine. It is a severe recurring headache, often starting in the teens, that usually affects one side of the head near the eye and is accompanied with nausea or vomiting. In what is called 'classical migraine', the headache is usually preceded by visual symptoms, such as flashing or coloured lights, or bright diagonal zigzags. Sometimes migraine can cause brief loss of speech or even temporary weakness or tingling down one side of the body. Attacks may last from minutes to hours but severe attacks force the sufferer to lie down in a quiet, darkened room until the headache disappears.

A tendency to migraine is often inherited. At least half the migraine sufferers can trace migraine, or another allergic condition, as an inherited family characteristic.

Migraine attacks can be triggered by all sorts of neotoxins, including:

- **Biological neotoxins**
  Food, fasting, dieting and irregular meals, all of which cause *hypoglycaemia*; chocolate, sweets and sugar, white flour, coffee, citrus fruits, cheese, alcohol especially red wine, onions, fried foods, tea, pork, seafood.
- **Chemical neotoxins**
  Intense smells and irritant chemicals; effect of hormones, especially in women and associated with menstrual cycle; oral contraception and other medication; smoking.
- **Physical neotoxins**
  EM and radiated energy, bright sunlight, glare, TV flicker, fluorescent lights, hot baths, loud noises.
- **Mental neotoxins**
  Stress, change in routine, e.g. holiday/ travel/shift work/sleep pattern, work change, excitement, tension, anger, depression, shock, exercise.

What causes migraine?

It is not known what causes migraine. The brain itself does not feel pain but the pain of migraine seems to originate from blood vessels surrounding the brain. The theories of how migraine is caused include:

- Presence of vasoactive amines (proteins that affect the size of arteries, e.g. like histamine) which cause blood vessels surrounding the brain to change in size and give pain. These vasoactive amines occur in food or are released by foods.

- Hypoglycaemia (low blood sugar) causes the blood vessels around the brain to dilate in order to increase blood flow and give the brain more sugar, which is its only source of energy.
- Allergies cause water retention throughout the body. If the brain retains water there is a problem because the brain is enclosed in a rigid skull and has nowhere to expand. Consequently, the blood vessels tend to get pushed flat and this is painful.

How can I cure migraine?

Once a qualified practitioner has excluded other important causes of headache, (e.g. head injury, high blood pressure and brain tumours), follow the guidelines to help your migraine. This advice is likely to assist about 2 out of 3 adult migraine sufferers and 9 out of 10 child migraine sufferers.

- Go on the Superhealth plan to reduce your total load of neotoxins;
- Identifying your food neotoxins by going on an exclusion diet (see page 000);
- Take regular meals and stop your blood sugar from dropping to low levels due to starvation. Avoid food and drinks containing large amounts of sugar, white flour or alcohol – all of which may cause reactive hypoglycaemia (see Chapter 10);
- For women, stop taking the oral contraceptive pill and *make alternative contraceptive arrangements*;
- Stop smoking and passive smoking (sitting next to someone who is smoking);
- Try to avoid loud noises and flashing lights (discos), and in bright sunlight wear high quality sunglasses to prevent glare;
- Avoid formaldehyde, chlorine, cleaning agents, solvents, glues and paints, smoke, exhaust fumes, natural gas and chlorine (see Chapter 3);
- Try to avoid stressful situations and get adequate sleep. Don't work shifts.

Migraine exclusion diet
Completely avoid the following:

All cheese
Dairy products especially cream
Coffee
White flour
All sugars and sweets
Chocolate and cocoa
Citrus fruits
Onions, chives, leeks and garlic
Tomatoes, bananas and avocado
Eggs
Seafood and pickled herrings
All mammal meat (beef, lamb and all forms of pork)
Fried foods
Yeast, vinegar, mushrooms and marmite
Tea
All alcohol drinks

NB. This is not a long-term diet, but merely an exclusion diet to identify the migraine producing food.

Suggested vitamin and mineral supplements for adults

Vitamin B_1	25 mg	daily
Vitamin B_2	25 mg	daily
Vitamin B_3	50 mg	daily
Vitamin B_5	50 mg	daily
Vitamin B_6	25 mg	daily
Vitamin C	2,000 mg	daily
Vitamin E	200 iu	daily
Magnesium	500 mg	daily
Zinc	15 mg	daily
Cod Liver Oil	10 ml	daily
Evening Primrose Oil	1,500 mg	daily

Drink 3 to 4 pints of bottled spring water a day.

Caution: These vitamin and mineral supplements should only be taken by patients who have received clearance from their own doctor.

EPILEPSY

This is a disease of the brain in which the normal rhythmic electrical activity is replaced by a concerted electrical discharge affecting the whole brain, which then causes unconsciousness and/or fits. There may be a brief warning or 'aura' before the start of the epilepsy, and after the fit there is usually a period of confusion with amnesia, headache and sleepiness.

Epilepsy affects 1 in 200 of the population, and frequently follows damage to the brain. This brain damage often occurs at birth due to pressure on the head, e.g. through using forceps or due to a reduced oxygen supply following a delay or difficulty in birth. Epilepsy can also occur later in life following a head injury or other brain insult, e.g. meningitis, stroke, brain tumour, pesticide exposure, and usually develops before the age of 20 years. However, having epilepsy does not necessarily mean that your mental abilities are limited. Well known sufferers from epilepsy include Leonardo de Vinci, Handel, Lord Byron and Van Gogh.

Any person can be made to have a fit if given enough of the wrong sort of stimulation, e.g. electroconvulsive therapy (ECT) which causes a fit in anyone after an electric current is passed through the substance of the brain. The threshold for a fit in the average person is high. In an epileptic, the threshold for a fit is much lower, due to previous brain damage and scarring of the brain's surface.

The following neotoxins can induce an epileptic fit:

- **Biological**
  Hypoglycaemia: This is induced by missing meals, dieting and starvation. Reactive hypoglycaemia is induced by a diet rich in sugar, white flour and alcohol.

  The other factors that may encourage fits are hormonal changes, e.g. those occurring in women during their menstrual cycle, excess body water, low sodium and calcium, and infections.
- **Chemicals**
  Missed anti-epileptic tablets; drugs and drug interactions; contraceptive pill; antidepressants; certain tranquillizers and drug withdrawal hallucinations; pesticides and fungicides, especially those applied to wood; and lead.
- **Physical**
  Light, especially flickering or flashing lights, e.g. TV, sun flickering through railings, other EM radiation, heat, cold and noise.
- **Mental**
  Stress, emotion, fear and anxiety, sleep disturbance.

What should I do if someone has an epileptic fit?

This is a relatively straightforward piece of first aid. You may get a little warning of the onset of the fit because the epileptic starts to behave oddly, with repetitive movements or actions for 20 to 30 seconds before the onset. Then you should try to:

- Catch them before they fall so that they don't strike their head. Place them flat on the ground on their side so that they don't inhale their own vomit, having first moved them to a safe place. The coma position prevents inhalation of vomit into the lungs.
- Cushion the head and loosen clothing. Do not restrict movement or put anything in the mouth.
- Take the pulse and ensure that the heart continues beating. During the fit the epileptic will probably *briefly* stop breathing and even go blue. However, providing the

heart continues beating, no extra treatment is necessary.

● If this is the first fit, it is important that the cause is investigated by a qualified person. Your account of the fit will be very useful, since the epileptic will have no recollection of it. The most common cause of a fit in an established epileptic, is missing their anti-epileptic tablets, and/or drinking alcohol, which causes reactive hypoglycaemia.

How can an epileptic reduce the risk of a fit or other problems?

● Use the Superhealth plan to reduce your total load of neotoxins by taking clean air, clean food and clean water. Be sure to take vitamin and mineral supplements including Vitamin A, Vitamin B complex, Vitamin C, Calcium, Magnesium and Manganese.

● Don't get overhungry, but take regular meals and avoid excessive intake of sugars and white flour;

● Don't drink more than 2 units of alcohol per day (1 unit = 1 measure of spirits, 1 glass of wine, half a pint of beer);

● Take your anti-epileptic medication as prescribed. If you can't remember if you've taken a dose it is probably better to take another one, but make a note that you've taken it;

● Avoid other drugs which may cause an interaction, e.g. antidepressants, anti-histamines, excess alcohol;

● Ideally, you should be on a single type of medicine to stop your epilepsy. Have the blood level of that medicine checked every 6 months to ensure that the dose that you are taking is neither too high or too low;

● Women hoping to become pregnant should take the medication least likely to cause malformations such as hare lip, cleft palate and spina bifida. Do not stop medication during pregnancy, since a mother having fits causes a risk of damage to the baby due to reduced oxygen supply;

● Avoid halocarbons, pesticides and lead (see Chapter 3);

● Avoid flashing lights, loud noises, and being close (within 100 yards) to high voltage power lines;

● Avoid stress, emotion and sleep disturbance;

● Don't swim or climb without supervision;

● Don't take a deep bath while alone in the house. Either take a shallow bath or a shower;

● Don't lock doors and, where possible, have doors that open outwards, (so that in the event of an epileptic fit you are not unconscious behind the door, jamming it shut);

● Fires and cookers should always be guarded;

● Sleep with a safety pillow or no pillow at all;

● Don't drive a car unless you have been free of a fit for 3 years. Unfortunately, any fits experienced over the age of 3 years, disqualifies a person from driving a Heavy Goods Vehicle or Public Services Vehicle for life;

● Wear an identity bracelet stating that you are epileptic and the tablets and dose taken.

MULTIPLE SCLEROSIS (MS)

This is a disease of the brain and spinal cord in which the nerve fibres stop working due to removal of the myelin layer (a fat) surrounding them. The underlying problem in MS is a failure of the nerves to conduct messages, since they have lost their insulation. This is rather like trying to have a telephone conversation using a cable with many wires in it, all of which have been stripped of insulation.

MS usually occurs in episodes, with periods

of recovery in between. Symptoms include:

paralysis
tingling and numbness
loss of vision
tremor

The recovery phase is usually not complete, and with each attack the whole picture usually gets a little worse. MS is more common in temperate climates, and 6 out of 10 people have their first attack between the ages of 20 and 40 years. It is slightly more common in women.

The cause of MS is not known but theories include:

- A 'slow' virus similar to the one that causes Mad Cow Disease (BSE);
- Long-term side-effect of mercury coming from amalgam dental fillings in the mouth;
- Other toxic metals such as aluminium, copper or lead;
- Other food and chemical neotoxins.

What can MS patients do to help themselves?

- Use the Superhealth plan to reduce your total load of neotoxins by getting clean air, clean food, and clean water.
- Consider having all dental amalgam fillings removed. The most dangerous fillings are the ones that act like tiny batteries and produce a high voltage within the mouth. You will need to consult an Environmental Medicine specialist in order to see if this is likely to help your case.
- Candida-free and gluten-free diets sometimes help MS.
- The vitamin and mineral supplements that help MS sufferers include Vitamin B complex and especially the essential fatty acids (fish oils and Evening Primrose oil), as well as the usual list that aids detoxification.

CHAPTER TWELVE

BEATING ANXIETY, DEPRESSION AND PSYCHIATRIC DISORDERS

Mental illness, especially in the minor forms, is alarmingly common. At least half of all GP consultations are directly or indirectly attributed to 'anxiety', 'depression' and many poorly defined mental symptoms such as 'no energy', 'irritability' and 'feeling off'. In fact a large proportion of these mental symptoms are due to allergies.

Unfortunately, due to the legacy given us by ancient philosophers, the mind and body are seen as separate entities. In reality they are inextricably linked, and any problem with one will cause a knock-on problem with the other. A large proportion of people with mental problems can be helped by:

● Reducing the total load of neotoxins by taking clean air, clean food and clean water;
● Removing the neotoxins to which they are sensitive;
● Taking *adequate* supplements of vitamins (especially B and C), minerals and other nutrients (especially folic acid).

The more common mental symptoms that can be made worse by environmental pollution include:

● Recurrent tiredness, weakness, fatigue, malaise and sleep irregularities;
● Poor co-ordination, dizziness and unsteadiness;

● Poor memory and concentration;
● Irritability, mood swings, personality changes, temper outbursts, restlessness.

The more common mental diseases that can be made worse by environmental pollution include:

Anxiety and panic attacks and agoraphobia
Depression and seasonal affective disorders
Dementia and confusion
Addiction – see Chapter 13
Mania
Schizophrenia

ANXIETY

How can I tell if I am suffering from anxiety?

This may not seem like a sensible question. However, many bodily symptoms can be caused by an anxious mind. In fact, every single system of the body can be affected by anxiety which itself can be induced by an allergic problem. If you have many of the symptoms below you may be suffering from anxiety and/or an allergy.

● **Heart and vessels:** palpitations, fast heart beat, rise in blood pressure, chest discomfort, fainting, pallor, flushing and sweating;

- **Lungs:** chest tightness, shortness of breath, hyperventilation;
- **Bowels:** dry mouth, indigestion, nausea, vomiting, abdominal pain, bloating, flatulence, weight loss, diarrhoea, constipation;
- **Genitourinary system:** frequency of urination, pain on urination, irregular, light or heavy periods, loss of sexual urge, impotence;
- **Musculoskeletal system:** aches and pains in muscles and joints, backache;
- **Nervous system – physical symptoms:** tremor, increased muscle tension, poor vision and hearing, weakness, giddiness, headaches, dilation of pupils;
- **Nervous system – mental symptoms:** worried and tearful about the future, irritability, tension, fatigue, emotional instability, irrational fear, difficulty in sleeping, poor memory and concentration, restlessness, very active mind.

To cope with anxiety, you should first be assessed by a qualified practitioner who must check that your problem is not due to a serious disease such as, thyroid problem, heart valve disease, a clot on the lungs, complication of diabetes, rare forms of epilepsy, tumours, or side-effects of medicines. Once these are excluded you may try the Superhealth Plan. You will need to avoid coffee, alcohol and sugar, and take adequate B vitamins, vitamins C and E, calcium, magnesium and zinc.

DEPRESSION

How can I tell if I am suffering from depression?

As with anxiety, bodily symptoms may be caused by a depressed mind. In a similar way every single system of the body can be affected by depression which itself can be induced by an allergic problem:

- **Heart and vessels:** sweating;
- **Lungs:** breathlessness;
- **Bowels:** dry mouth, loss of appetite, indigestion, constipation, weight gain;
- **Genitourinary system:** irregular or heavy/light periods, painful periods, reduced sexual interest;
- **Musculoskeletal system:** joint pain, low backache, slouching when walking;
- **Nervous system – physical:** headache, monotonous voice, tremor, slow body movement;
- **Nervous system – mental:** sad, regretful or guilty about the past, self-neglect, hopelessness, guilt, worthlessness, obsessions, paranoid attacks, loss of self-confidence, early morning wakening, loss of pleasure in any activity, loss of energy, tiredness, inability to make decisions, suicidal thoughts.

Before deciding that you have depression, you must see a qualified practitioner who must exclude other causes for depression, including diseases such as myxoedema, vitamin B_{12} deficiency, diabetes, alcohol toxicity, drug addiction, side-effects of prescribed drugs, industrial exposure to toxic chemicals and metals e.g. mercury, head injury, heart disease and raised blood pressure.

Depression is more likely to occur after critical times in life, and after negative life events, i.e.:

puberty
marital breakdown
pregnancy
loss of job
menopause
moving house
retirement
disablement
death of spouse.

195

Having little money, being unemployed, having poor housing or education and many dependants make depression more likely.

After you have excluded other problems you can use the Superhealth plan to treat depression. You will need to take B vitamins, together with some biotin and folic acid, vitamins C and E, calcium and magnesium, potassium and evening primrose oil.

CAN I HELP MY ELDERLY RELATIVE WITH DEMENTIA?

Dementia is due to a progressive loss of memory and intellect. It is more common in old people. Symptoms include:

- Poor *short term* memory – memories of childhood unimpaired but no ability to remember the events of the previous day;
- Slow in doing things, especially in *new* situations, e.g. using a new gadget;
- Increasing difference between what the person *says* and they actually *do*;
- Confusion and disorientation in place and time may occur;
- Deterioration in behaviour and conforming to social convention (i.e. walking in the street in their pyjamas).

Dementia is a situation where other illness must be ruled out by a qualified practitioner. These problems include, myxoedema, vitamin deficiency (especially B_3 and B_{12}) diabetes, alcohol toxicity, drug addiction, side-effects of prescribed drugs, industrial exposure to toxic chemicals and metals, e.g. mercury, head injury, heart disease and raised blood pressure, and depression.

Once the diseases have been excluded, the Superhealth plan may be tried and sometimes can produce a large improvement.

CAN ENVIRONMENTAL MEDICINE HELP SCHIZOPHRENIA?

Schizophrenia is a serious mental disorder in which the patient has little or no insight into his/her condition (a psychosis). The symptoms include:

- Delusions and hallucinations;
- Feeling as though voices were talking about and controlling him/her;
- Impulsive actions and bizarre behaviour;
- Difficulty with personal relationships.

Despite being a mental illness, there is no doubt that some cases of schizophrenia are due to allergies, often wheat allergy, and occur due to the inability of that person's body to work properly on their existing diet. Strong evidence that schizophrenia is due to a chemical problem is the fact that blood is taken from a schizophrenic person and transfused into a normal person (of the same blood group), it causes the appearance of schizophrenic-like symptoms in the previously normal person.

In some cases, modification of the diet and addition of large doses of vitamins, minerals and other nutrients is able to cure schizophrenia. *This treatment should only be carried out under the supervision of a suitably qualified person.*

CHAPTER THIRTEEN

THE ADDICTIONS – SMOKING, ALCOHOL, COFFEE, TEA AND CHOCOLATE

Addictions are the commonest cause of *preventable* ill health in the western world. Addictions can be defined as a difficulty in stopping taking a neotoxin because of cravings and withdrawal symptoms which develop in the absence of the substance.

The common sources of addiction include neotoxins such as:

- Nicotine from smoking;
- Alcohol from alcoholic beverages;
- Caffeine from coffee, chocolate, cola, tea;
- Sugar – causing reactive hypoglycaemia;
- Other foods, especially junk foods containing additives (E numbers);
- Chemicals, including solvents, paints, and glues, petrochemicals, halocarbons, aerosols;
- Prescribed drugs, e.g. benzodiazepines, barbiturates;
- Non-prescribed drugs.

Owing to the vast increase in the number of chemicals in the environment, addictions are becoming more rather than less common.

Addiction is a form of allergy. The craving for an addicted substance is one of the classic symptoms. Most addictive substances are actually poisons (neotoxins), which, in small doses, initially have the ability to give a 'lift', 'buzz' or euphoria, but in larger doses have the opposite effect and cause sedation. The greater the magnitude and faster the onset of the euphoria, the greater the likelihood that a substance will become addictive. For example, cigarettes very rapidly give a big lift (within 7 seconds), and in a short time often become an unshakeable habit. However, almost any neotoxin can become addictive if taken for long enough and frequently enough, especially if it is a fat soluble chemical which enables it to get rapidly into the brain.

An addict continuously taking a neotoxin goes through the three stages of the general adaption syndrome (see page 33). The first stage is the 'alarm phase' in which the subject immediately feels unwell. This occurs with the first exposure, e.g. first cigarette or first glass of alcohol.

If exposure continues, the subject rapidly passes into the second stage of 'adaption' (or 'resistance'). In this stage each exposure gives a 'buzz' or a 'lift', which is followed by a withdrawal reaction (which feels like a hangover). As a good general rule the higher the initial lift, the more severe the ensuing hangover; this is an effect called *Bipolarity*. In addition, when the levels of lift and depression are small, symptoms tend to be localized to one organ. However, as the swings become larger, symptoms become generalized, especially affecting the brain and depressing or elevating mood. Consequently, injected or inhaled heroin which gives an enormous initial 'lift' is followed by debilitating depression and even semi-coma.

If exposure to the addictive neotoxin continues, a process called 'habituation' or 'tolerance' occurs. In this state the body reacts less to each exposure, and is able to break down the neotoxin more quickly, due to activation of the enzymes that metabolize it. This results in the subject taking higher and more frequent doses in order to produce the same 'lift'. The phenomenon of habituation or tolerance is well recognized by smokers, drinkers and addicts who have to step up their intake to avoid the unpleasant withdrawal symptoms. At this stage, many addicts will totally deny that they are addicted, since exposure to the addictive neotoxin actually makes them feel well ('masked allergy'). This addiction is 'unmasked' by withdrawing the addictive neotoxin and precipitating the withdrawal reaction of hangover and craving.

The withdrawal reaction can be 'turned off' in two ways:

- Taking another usual sized dose of the addictive neotoxin. This will, of course, produce a further withdrawal reaction when it wears off.
- Taking a tiny micro-dose, either by mouth or injected by hypodermic needle into the skin. This micro-dose needs to be very dilute, and although the theory is unclear, appears to work in an electrical way rather like homoeopathy. The micro-dose is often able to stop the withdrawal hangover and craving. A typical turnoff dose might be 1 part in 100,000 or part in 1 million but will only work for 24 to 48 hours before a further micro-dose is required. If used under medical supervision, this micro-dose can be used to help most addictions.

If exposure to the addictive neotoxin continues, then the subject passes through a 'transitional' stage, in which even more frequent and larger doses of neotoxin are needed to produce a 'lift', which is rapidly followed by more profound and persistent hangovers. In the transition stage the subject feels unwell most of the day. This is rapidly followed by the third stage of 'exhaustion'.

In the 'exhaustion' stage, each exposure to the addictive neotoxin gives an immediate unpleasant reaction and the 'lift' or 'buzz' effect of the addictive neotoxin is lost. The subject feels ill all the time and the amount of neotoxin tolerated drops dramatically. In this stage cross-sensitivity to many other substances is common, as is total allergy syndrome, in which the immune system becomes very non-selective, responding to almost everything.

What factors encourage addiction?

Several factors have an influence on the addiction process.

A genetic predisposition

The more members of a family who have allergic illnesses and symptoms, the more likely that addiction will occur.

A high dose of the addictive neotoxin

The higher the dose, the greater the risk of addiction. A massive dose, such as occurs with exposure to a chemical spill, is likely permanently to alter the susceptibility to addiction.

Frequent exposure to the addictive neotoxin

Frequent exposures increase the risk of addiction. If a substance is taken frequently (more than every 3 days), then it is likely to cause addiction. This is more common if a substance is easily available (e.g. alcohol, controlled drugs to medical professions), and if there is strong social pressure to take a substance (e.g. if all friends are smokers). The longer the time that a substance has been taken overall, the more likely that it will lead to addiction.

The way that the addictive neotoxin is taken

The faster that the addictive neotoxin gets to the brain (where the addictive process occurs), the more likely that it will become addictive. The slowest route (and least addictive route), is by mouth. Much faster and more addictive is intravenous injection, where an injected substance will reach the brain in 15 seconds. Even faster and by far the most addictive method is inhalation (e.g. smoking, 'glue sniffing', crack smoking), in which case addictive neotoxins reach the brain in 7 seconds.

If the substance produces euphoria

The higher the 'lift' or 'buzz', the greater the powers of addiction.

Combination of substances

For example, foods are more addictive if taken with alcohol or other fat soluble substances that can easily enter the brain.

Age, general health and mental state

The younger, fitter and better mentally adjusted you are, the less likely that you will become addicted.

Your total load of neotoxins

The greater your total load of neotoxins (biological, chemical, physical and mental), the greater the likelihood of addiction.

What are the common withdrawal symptoms of addiction?

All systems of the body are affected by withdrawal symptoms caused by removing an addictive neotoxin. Symptoms include:

- **Heart and blood vessels:** palpitations, rapid heartbeats, sweating;
- **Lungs:** difficulty in breathing;
- **Bowels:** appetite loss, weight gain or weight loss, dry mouth, nausea, vomiting, abdominal cramp, diarrhoea;
- **Genitourinary system:** incontinence, frequency of urination;
- **Skin:** rashes and urticaria, itching and goose flesh;
- **Musculoskeletal:** muscular and joint aches, lower back pain;
- **Nervous system – physical:** fever, headache, muscle twitching, muscle weakness, runny nose, tremors, unsteady gait, visual problem;
- **Nervous system – mental:** anxiety, concentration problems, craving, delirium, depression, dizziness, drowsiness, fatigue unrelieved by rest, hallucinations, hyperactivity, insomnia, irritability, malaise, temporary insanity, tremor.

It is important to realize that addiction is very idiosyncratic. A drug that is addictive to most people is not addictive to all. Also, personal immunity from addiction to one drug does not mean that you will have immunity to another.

HOW CAN I BEAT ADDICTION TO NICOTINE?

Nicotine addiction takes about 2 to 3 years to develop fully. After this time the addiction to nicotine can be as strong as an addiction to heroin. The nicotine can have a stimulating or sedating effect, depending upon the type of smoking used. Short puffs with many gaps causes stimulation of the brain but long deep puffs causes a sedating effect on the brain. A nicotine addict smokes in a way designed to get the desired degree of stimulation or sedation.

Your stop smoking plan

1. There are three stages. Choose strategies from the following pages you would like to use to help yourself stop smoking.
2. Choose a day two to three weeks ahead, make a note yourself, and tell other people that you are going to give up smoking on that day.
3. Enlist the support of others, and avoid trigger factors and trigger behaviour.

Look at the following lines of alternatives to select strategies and activities that will assist you, underlining those you intend to use.

For people who want to give up completely

- **Identify the problems which cause you to continue smoking.**
- **Remove the trigger factors and trigger behaviour**
  Change your routine and avoid or reduce all factors and behaviour that trigger smoking, such as stress, anger, coffee or alcohol (try tonic water instead), and social situations and parties with other smokers (don't accept cigarettes!). Avoid personal crises, stressful holidays and contact with other smokers in the early stages.
- **Find substitutes for smoking**
  These may be either activities or objects. Exercise, especially breathing exercises, and social contact will divert your attention away from smoking, and there are many activities that can keep the hands or the mouth busy, such as toothpicks, mouth-washes and chewing mints or gum. Go for

a walk after a meal. Take a shower before breakfast and a warm bath at night.
- **Gain mental and emotional support from yourself and others**
  Mentally prepare yourself to give up smoking by setting some date in advance, then tell others. Overcome your fears and objections to stopping smoking. See yourself as a non-smoker. Don't apologize for not smoking. Ask friends and relatives to help you through the withdrawal symptoms.
- **Reward yourself for non-smoking behaviour.**
  For example, put aside the money saved from smoking for some other non-smoking (preferably non-fattening) treat.

For smokers who wish to give up gradually

- **Make it more difficult to smoke**
  Make your cigarettes and/or lighter less accessible by hiding them, putting them in a drawer, pocket or another room. Some smokers try the nuisance approach of changing brands with every new pack, and putting out a cigarette after each puff, or else leaving it in the ashtray. Others do not let themselves smoke while doing another activity, for example, watching television, eating, reading or drinking, and if they wish to smoke they must stop the other activity. Other smokers make certain rooms or times non-smoking and deliberately go to places where smoking is not allowed, e.g. sitting in the non-smoking part of a bus, train or restaurant.
- **Employ delaying tactics**
  Increase the time between cigarettes: one hour in the first week, two hours in the second week, and so on. Cut out the 'easy' cigarettes first, by not smoking before breakfast or one hour before bedtime, and

gradually increase the non-smoking period.

- **Reduce the dose of nicotine**
Smoke only half a cigarette and do not inhale. Ration yourself to a certain number of cigarettes a day, or try a pipe or cigar but don't inhale. Change to a lower nicotine content cigarette, and allow only one cigarette after a meal or one cigarette per hour. Drink lots of water to flush out the nicotine. Smokers will need to take large amounts of Vitamin C together with adequate B Vitamins, Vitamin E, magnesium, zinc, selenium and essential fatty acids.

HOW CAN I BEAT ADDICTION TO ALCOHOL?

Alcoholism may be an addiction to:

- Alcohol;
- Yeast;
- The food from which the alcohol was fermented, (e.g. grapes – brandy, cane sugar – rum, barley-malt – whisky). Many alcoholics who stop drinking alcohol continue to stimulate their addiction by continuing to take the food from which the drink is made, e.g. rum drinking alcoholics who give up rum but still take cane sugar.

As well as allergy, excessive intake of alcohol is strongly associated with many other diseases, including cirrhosis of the liver, inflammation of the stomach, numerous cancers, diabetes, epilepsy, brain failure and psychiatric problems. Excessive alcohol intake is a major cause of ill health, and one in seven hospital admissions is for an alcohol-related disease. The majority of road traffic accidents, many relationship problems and much violent crime are wholly or partly due to alcohol.

You should consider reducing or giving up alcohol if you:

- Drink more than 21 units a week for men (14 units a week for women);
- Drink more than twice a day or four times a week;
- Have one of the above disease or problems;
- Take a drug that interacts with alcohol, for example, tranquillizers, antidepressants, pain-killers;
- Hope to start a family (men or women);
- Are pregnant.

A reasonable target for alcohol intake, if it is equally spread over the week, is a maximum of 14 units per week for men and 10 units per week for women. If you feel that you drink too much, here are some strategies that will probably help you:

- Try to decide why you drink too much. Is it due to emotion e.g. tension, anger, frustration, depression or happiness? If so, then deal with the underlying problem.
- Decide where you drink too much, and change your routine to avoid these places.
- Change your social life, and avoid your previous drinking partner(s). Examine your drinking pattern: see if you drink regularly every day, or just binge occasionally. Try to reduce the number of times you drink and the overall amount.
- Admit to yourself that you drink too much alcohol (or even that you are an alcoholic), and decide that you definitely want to give up completely (the best strategy). Failing that, decide to reduce your intake to a safe level.
- If you do find yourself in a pub, try a non-alcoholic drink, or else change to a different low-alcoholic drink. Don't buy rounds, and reduce the volume by drinking half measures.
- Have an excuse ready to explain why you are not drinking, for example, 'I'm driving home, I'm saving money/losing weight,

going out to dinner afterwards, had too much to drink last night, on the wagon, doctor's orders.'
- Get expert help from your GP, or consult Alcoholics Anonymous – the local telephone number is in your phone book.

To combat addiction to alcoholism it is important to take high levels of all the B Vitamins, together with folic acid and biocin, choline and inositol, also Vitamins A, C and E, magnesium, zinc, selenium and evening primrose oil.

HOW CAN I BEAT CAFFEINE ADDICTION?

Caffeine is a powerful stimulant. It is present in many drinks and foods, and some medications including:

> Coffee
> Tea
> Cola soft drinks
> Chocolate
> Many analgesics

It is very common to get withdrawal symptoms, including a severe headache, 1 to 3 days after removing caffeine from the diet. Caffeine addiction can be beaten by using the Superhealth plan, and completely avoiding all sources of caffeine.

HOW CAN I BEAT SUGAR ADDICTION?

Follow Chapter 10 and go onto a low-sugar, low processed-carbohydrate diet, also avoiding alcohol.

HOW CAN I BEAT ADDICTIONS CAUSED BY OTHER FOODS?

Follow the Superhealth plan in Chapter 6.

HOW CAN I BEAT CHEMICAL ADDICTIONS?

Follow Chapter 3 to find out which chemical(s) you are allergic to. Then completely avoid exposure to that substance and similar related substances as further described in Chapter 3. Take plenty of Vitamin C (4,000 mg for adults). Lower your fat consumption and especially avoid red meat, which, because of the high fat content, sometimes contains chemicals. Instead, take organic cold-pressed oils to build up your essential fatty acids.

HOW CAN I BEAT ADDICTION TO PRESCRIBED MEDICINES?

You must do this in conjunction with the doctor who is prescribing your tablets. Go onto the Superhealth plan to reduce your total load of neotoxins. After you have done this, your general health will probably improve considerably and you may no longer need your medication. You must, however, let your doctor make this decision and then you can reduce the number of tablets you take gently.

HOW CAN I BEAT ADDICTION TO NON-PRESCRIBED DRUGS?

To do this you also need to go on the Superhealth plan. Also you must:
- Make a decision for lifelong abstinence;
- Throw away all stores of drugs and equipment for taking them;
- Change your social life, avoiding other drug-takers and people who supply drugs;
- Enlist support from family, friends and doctor.

CHAPTER FOURTEEN

CHILDREN'S HEALTH PROBLEMS

Almost every child in the western world will suffer from some sort of allergic problem at some time. The peak age for development of allergies is 0 to 2 years. At this young age both the immune and detoxification systems and the bowels are immature. Consequently, allergies are much more likely to occur, especially after a trigger factor such as infection, usually a bowel infection, or teething.

WHICH FACTORS WILL MAKE MY CHILD MORE LIABLE TO SUFFER FROM AN ALLERGY?

Genetic predisposition

Having one allergic parent increases the likelihood of a child suffering allergies. Having both parents who are prone to allergies increases the risk still further.

Genetically induced allergies occur because the body produces either poorly functioning enzymes or insufficient enzymes (e.g. asthma, cystic fibrosis, coeliac disease).

A high total load of neotoxins

Neotoxins may come from biological, chemical, physical or mental sources. A high total load of neotoxins reduces general health.

Infections

Infections, especially viral and fungal infections that damage the bowel wall, allow undigested foods and other potentially dangerous substances to enter the bloodstream, where they may overwhelm the immature immune and detoxification systems.

A deficient immune system

The baby's immune system must start protecting the body from infection immediately after birth. Up until birth, maternal antibodies can enter the baby's bloodstream via the placenta. These maternal antibodies last until the infant is about 6 months old. After birth, the breast feeding mother can continue to give her baby antibodies in breast milk. These antibodies help the baby fight infection and can neutralize infections within the gut. Bottle fed children taking cow's milk do not receive this immune system boost.

The immune system can be deficient due to hereditary reasons, premature birth, depression of the immune system due to any neotoxin (drugs, infection or poisoning), vitamin and mineral deficiency, or any other disease affecting general health (e.g. heart, lung, kidney or liver disease).

Mother's poor diet

Breast milk tends to concentrate foods and chemicals found in the mother's body. If the

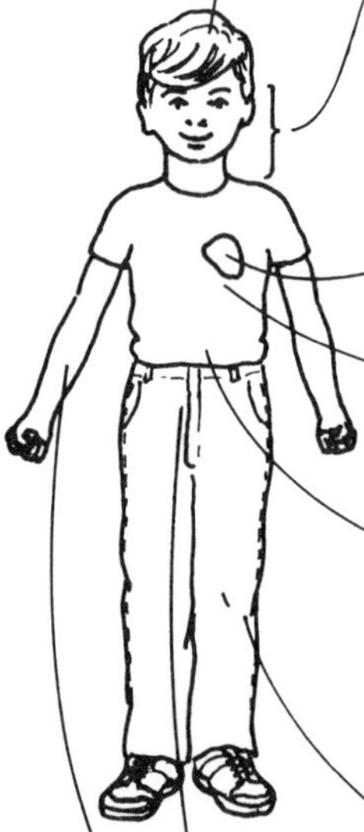

Localized symptoms

Brain Symptoms
physical: headaches, fits and giddiness, poor vision, hearing and coordination
behavioural: overactive or underactive, addictions
thought and learning: poor memory and concentration

Eyes, Face and Ears, Nose and Throat
glassy eyes, shadows and wrinkles under eyes and nose, blocked, running and itching eyes, ears, nose and throat, sneezing and sniffing

Heart
palpatations and fast pulse

Lung
asthma, breathlessness, wheezing

Alimentary Canal
excessive thirst, feeding difficulties, abdominal pains and bloating, constipation, diarrhoea, flatulence

Bones and Joints
arthritis, rheumatism

Skin
eczeme, red and itching rashes, urticaria

Genito-urinary
bed wetting, cystitis, thrush

Generalized symptoms

during pregnancy highly active in womb

failure to grow

tired all the time

fatigue

muscular weakness

swelling of many parts of the body, including eyelids, lips and mouth, hands and fingers, abdomen and ankles

sweating (intermittent)

overweight, underweight or having a rapidly changing weight

recurrent infections

Figure 14.1 **Common symptoms seen in the allergic child**

mother has a poor diet, repetitive in commonly allergic foods (e.g. eggs, milk, wheat) and also high in chemicals (e.g. from smoking or drinking), then the baby is more likely to develop an allergy.

Early weaning and repetitive diet

If breast feeding is stopped too early (before 6 months) and highly allergenic cows milk feed or other allergens (dairy products, eggs, white, chocolate, food additives) are given to the child every day, then an allergy is much more likely to develop.

WHAT ARE THE SYMPTOMS OF CHILDHOOD ALLERGY?

The most notable thing about allergies is the *variety* of the symptoms, which may affect *all* systems. As the American College of Allergists has said, 'Allergies do not do everything but they can do anything.' The commonest symptoms to be found in an allergic child are:

- During pregnancy baby highly active in the womb;
- Baby very thirsty especially at breakfast (drinks 1 pint or more of fluid);
- Feeding difficulties (regurgitation, vomiting, won't take food despite being hungry);
- Failure to grow (see child Ht/Wt tables page 235 in Appendix);
- Abdominal pain, usually colic in nature, and bloating;
- Diarrhoea and/or constipation;
- 'Glassy' eyes as if in a trance;
- Dark blue, black or red shadows and/or wrinkles under the eyes;
- Sneezing and sniffing with runny, itchy or congested nose and eyes;
- Perception problems (can't see, hear or understand properly);

- Muscle and co-ordination problems. Constantly active with wriggling legs, hands or arms;
- Behaviour problems especially *sudden variations* in behaviour often after eating/drinking or exposure to a chemical;
- Thought and learning difficulties.

Every single system of the body can be affected by allergies. Surprisingly, allergy can make an organ or system overactive or underactive, the main finding being that it doesn't work as normal.

OTHER ALLERGIC DISEASES AND SYMPTOMS (LISTED BY SYSTEM)

Heart and circulation

Palpitations, changes in pulse rate, excessive sweating especially at night, changes in skin colour and temperature (slight fever), cold hands and feet, fluid retention.

Lungs, eyes, nose and ears

Itching eyes and nose, hay fever, allergic rhinitis, nose rubbing, snuffly, catarrh, post-nasal drip, recurrent sinusitis, bad breath, tonsillitis, glue ears, consistent throat clearing, hiccough, persistent cough, especially at night on exertion, breathlessness, asthma, recurrent infections of any of above organs.

Bowels

Itching mouth and throat, dribbling, recurrent mouth ulcers, always hungry, poor appetite and weight gain, underweight or overweight, faddy eater, food craving, prefers junk foods, nausea, colic and other abdominal pains, abdominal distension, frequent loose stool, flatulence, constipation.

Genitourinary system

Bed wetting, urinary incontinence, 'cystitis', thrush, vulvo-vaginitis.

Skin

Rashes, dry skin, cradle cap, eczema, dermatitis, itchy skin, hives and urticaria, dandruff.

Muscles and joints

Limb and especially leg pains, joint pains, joint twitching and stiffness, arthritis and muscular weakness.

Nervous system (physical)

Frequent headaches, migraine, fits and convulsions, blackouts, giddiness, very ticklish, does not feel pain, ME-type symptoms.

Perception problems: usual hearing problems. Muscle coordination problems: clumsy, poor muscle control.

Nervous system (psychological)

Behaviour problems: overactive

Endless energy, never tires (even after 16 hours), requires little sleep, wakes early, insomnia and nightmares, constantly in motion, fidgets, will not sit still. Aggression, hostility, irritability, excitable, impulsive, impatient, disobedient, disruptive, destructive, cannot be disciplined, uncooperative. Not aware of danger, always fighting, spitting, biting, kicking, hitting, pinching and pushing, cruel to other children and pets, abusive (temper tantrums and mood swings), vulgarity. Always breaking things, compulsively touching things.

Behaviour problems: underactive

Unhappy, whingeing, cries frequently, demanding, intolerant of delay or disappointment, wants immediate gratification, panics easily. Depression, (constantly tired, no energy, fatigue, malaise, exhausted). Difficulty in waking in morning for feeds, persistent yawning, requires excessive sleep or rest, extra-sensitive to loud noises, not aware of danger.

Thought and learning problems

Poor memory and concentration, short attention span, butterfly mind, poor comprehension, poor development/late with milestones, confusion, dyslexia, handwriting difficulties (large with hyperactivity and small with depression), doesn't know left from right, or up from down.

What foods most commonly cause food allergy in children and what substitutes can I use?

The foods that most commonly cause food allergy include cows' milk and dairy products (especially cheese), eggs, fish, wheat products (especially white flour), sugar, artificial colourings and additives (E numbers) and flavourings, soya products, tomato and citrus fruits. The best cows' milk substitutes for infants are Pregestamil and Nutramiten. For older children (over 6 months) goats' milk or ewes' milk can be used as a substitute for cows' milk although cross-sensitivity with these other milks sometimes appears. In order to get over the increased risk of infection in the goats' and ewes' milk, it is wise to boil them first. This has the added advantage of reducing the likelihood of allergic reactions since the size of the milk molecule is broken down by boiling, but the disadvantage of making the milk go off more quickly because its natural anti-bacterial activity is destroyed. Soya milk is another helpful cows' milk substitute, but may cause an allergic reaction itself.

Cows' milk can cause food allergy reaction

in two ways. The first is due to deficiency of the enzyme lactase, which breaks down the sugar lactose in the milk. This is a common temporary problem after damage to the intestinal wall from bowel infections. The second sort of cows' milk allergy is an allergy to the cows' milk protein, and this is usually a more long-term problem. Lactase deficiency usually causes diarrhoea, whereas cows' milk protein allergy causes a wide variety of symptoms. However both types are usually cured by exclusion of milk between 1 week and 6 months.

How do I stop my infant from becoming allergic?

There are several measures that will greatly reduce your infant's risk of becoming allergic.

- Don't smoke or drink alcohol during pregnancy; rotate foods (preferably organic) and drink bottled spring water. Take vitamin and mineral supplements and restrict your intake of allergenic foods like coffee and chocolate.
- Breast feed your child exclusively after birth, as even one bottle of cows' milk formula feed can increase the risk of allergy quite considerably. Continue to rotate your organic foods, drinking bottled spring water, and don't smoke or drink alcohol. The reason that it is important not to smoke is that the chemicals from the tobacco smoke are concentrated into the breast milk, which is then given to baby. If you are breast feeding, continue to restrict your intake of allergenic foods like coffee and chocolate.
- Do not wean baby from breast feeding until at least six months and leave common allergic foods like milk, wheat, eggs, tomatoes, chocolate and nuts until as late as possible in the diet. Try and leave wheat

until at least 9 months, eggs until a year, chocolate and nuts until two years. Wherever possible, give the child only organic food and restrict intake of food additives and sugar.

- Keep a notebook of food given to baby and add just one new food at a time to see if there is any reaction. Start with a small amount of food to be tested (one teaspoonful on the first day) and work up to a full portion over a week. Stop if you notice an allergic reaction. If your child has a bowel infection keep her or him on just spring water for a couple of days, to rest the bowel and prevent sensitivity to foods from developing.
- Try not to take any medication at all while you are breast feeding, as it will be a burden to baby's immune and detoxification system. There are some drugs which you definitely should not be taking while you are breast feeding, and whenever your doctor is going to give you medication you should always mention that you are feeding so that inappropriate drugs will not be used.
- Keep pets out of the house for the first six months of baby's life. This reduces the baby's exposure to other animal proteins and fur.
- Keep as many chemicals out of the house as possible (e.g. paints, glues, cleaners) and try to avoid anaesthetics for the first two years of life.

How can I help my baby's colic?

Colic is an intermittent abdominal pain caused by excess gas stretching the bowel. It usually comes on for about 30 seconds during which time baby draws up his legs to his chest; the pain then goes for about the same length of time before restarting. It may occur after foods, and if bottle fed you should suspect cows' milk or soya milk. If breast fed, then suspect the food that the mother has eaten in the previous 24 hours. Colic may occur due to over-feeding baby, especially first thing in the morning. The colic may occur because some milk passes into the lower bowel before all the lactose has been absorbed, thus causing gas production.

Can my baby's failure to thrive be due to allergy?

Failure to thrive has many causes, one of which is allergy. If your child is not gaining weight as expected then it is essential to get medical attention without delay. Common non-allergic causes include feeding problems, vomiting, malabsorption, diarrhoea, infection of the chest, ear or kidney, heart, kidney, liver, thyroid or brain problems. Common allergic problems causing failure to thrive include milk and other food allergies, coeliac disease, cystic fibrosis and lactose and sucrose sugar intolerances.

Can diet help conditions like coeliac disease and cystic fibrosis?

These are both congenital abnormalities, and the latter has been shown to be due to a defective gene which is inherited. Coeliac disease can be fully controlled by dietary measures and cystic fibrosis can be helped to a moderate degree. The problem in coeliac disease is that the small bowel lining is damaged by exposure to the protein gluten, which occurs in wheat. When gluten is taken in the diet it causes diarrhoea and mal-absorption and later in life it may cause a skin condition called dermatitis herpetiformis. Coeliac disease can be completely controlled by removing gluten from the diet. In cystic fibrosis, which occurs in approximately one in 2,000 births, the body makes mucus that is too

viscous and this will not drain from the lungs and pancreas with consequent problems with the function of these organs. Cystic fibrosis can be helped by taking oral digestive enzymes together with a diet high in essential fatty acids, vitamins and minerals and also clean air, clean food and a high intake of clean water.

Could my child's frequent infections be caused by allergy?

If the immune and detoxification systems are depressed by a high daily level of neotoxins (food additives, chemicals, drugs) and there is a deficiency of vitamins and minerals, then recurrent infections are more common. A fully functioning metabolism gives the body a high resistance to invasion by infections. One simple measure that can often help children suffering from recurrent chest and ear infections is to remove milk and milk products from the diet. This causes the body to make a less viscous mucus which drains more easily and is less likely to become infected.

Is cot death caused by an allergy?

Cot death or sudden infant death syndrome (SIDS) is an unexplained death of an infant under two years, and in Britain is the commonest cause of death in children between 1 and 12 months. Worryingly, it is becoming more rather than less common, affecting approximately one in every 500 births. The precise cause is not known; however, the known risk factors include: premature birth; maternal drug abuse and smoking; being a twin or a triplet; sleeping in a prone position with excessive blankets; having a single parent family and being illegitimate; being of low social class or having unemployed parents; being male; having a large number of brothers or sisters; and being in a bedroom heated all night in winter. The explanations that have been suggested to explain cot deaths include an allergy to milk protein, congenital lack of an enzyme, low blood glucose, or most recently, increasing levels of pesticide in food and consequently mother's milk, and also fungicides applied to babies' mattresses during manufacture. The rise in the use of pesticides on food has paralleled the rise in cot deaths, but extra evidence to suggest the role of pesticides is that cot death babies have been found to have poor control of their autonomic nervous system. This poor control of the autonomic nervous system, that controls blood pressure, pulse and waking is a condition that follows with pesticide poisoning. Cot death has also been associated with strong electromagnetic fields both in the radio and microwave bands. Cot deaths are unknown in some third world countries where the infants routinely sleep with their parents.

Can dyslexia and learning difficulties be allergic?

If your child has a *variable* dyslexia and difficulty in learning, then it is quite likely the problem is allergic. Similar problems that are *constant* are less likely to be amenable to treatment with exclusion diets, chemical exclusion and vitamin and mineral supplements. Adequate vitamin and mineral supplementation and exclusion of sugar and additives from a diet can certainly reduce aggressive behaviour and it is likely that similar measures may be able to increase IQ.

Can hyperactivity in children be caused by allergy?

A large proportion of hyperactive children can be greatly assisted by using principles of Environmental Medicine. Boys are affected three times more commonly than girls, and any hyperactive child may suffer any of the allergic symptoms listed on page 204. The target organ worst affected is the brain, and the most typical symptoms are constant movement, inability to sit still, aggression and disruption, inability to concentrate or learn at school, impatience, frustration, poor discipline and coordination, and difficulties with speech, hearing and vision.

The following exclusion diet helps quite a high proportion of hyperactive children. However, it must be emphasized that this is only a diagnostic diet *for short-term use*, and its function is to find the allergic foods. The food exclusion and challenge should be carried out as described on page 42.

Exclusion Diet for Hyperactivity

All milk and milk products, especially cheese and eggs
All mammal meats (beef, pork and lamb)
All processed meats – sausage, ham, salami, frankfurters
All wheat and wheat products
Barley, oats and rye
Tomatoes and citrus fruit
Onions
Chocolate
Sugar, yeast, vinegar and mushrooms
Smoked foods
Alcohol
All additives (E numbers and flavourings)
Soft drinks
Tea and coffee

Some children do react to salicylates and will also need to remove the following salicylate containing fruits:

Almonds, apples, apricots, blackberries, cherries, cucumbers, currants, gooseberries, grapes, lemons, oranges, peaches, plums, raspberries, strawberries, satsumas, tangerines, tomatoes.

What vitamin and mineral supplements will help hyperactivity?

The vitamin, mineral and other supplements necessary include Vitamin A, Vitamin B complex, Vitamin C, Vitamin E, calcium, magnesium, zinc, seleniun, manganese and chromium, together with evening primrose oil. The dose given depends on the age, weight and degree of illness in the child.

Why should I give my child vitamin and mineral supplements?

Unfortunately, vitamin and mineral deficiencies are increasingly common in children, due to a diet which is deficient in these essential nutrients and high in chemicals (like food additives) that use up or bind such vitamins and minerals. Before starting even a short-term exclusion diet in children, it is wise to give vitamin and mineral supplements, and these are essential when a child is on a long-term exclusion diet. An exclusion diet may paradoxically increase vitamin and mineral requirements, for example, when milk is excluded from the diet of a child who is allergic to milk normal growth rates often restart, with a consequent big increase in the demand for calcium.

How can I treat asthma, eczema, migraine and colitis?

See relevant chapters.

CHAPTER FIFTEEN

WOMEN'S HEALTH PROBLEMS

Women are about twice as likely to suffer from allergic illness as men. There are many reasons for this difference, including the following factors:

- The effect of the female hormone oestrogen: most allergic reactions cause the tissues involved to retain water. Oestrogen also causes water retention, increasing that already caused by the allergic reaction.

- The effect of the menstrual cycle on gut permeability: the hormone changes occurring immediately before a period (see page 218) make a woman's bowel more permeable to food. This extra permeability increases the incidence of allergies at this time, an effect known as the pre-menstrual syndrome (PMS). The hormonal part of this syndrome is caused by the falling level of progesterone, which causes less cortisone to be secreted by the adrenals, which in turn has a depressive effect on the immune and detoxification systems.

- The effect of pregnancy on allergies: during pregnancy, the level of the female hormone progesterone is very high and the metabolic rate is increased to provide the growing baby with nutrients and remove waste products. These changes make the woman's body more sensitive to common food allergens like milk, coffee and alcohol.

These increased sensitivities may disappear after pregnancy, but sometimes are permanent. Immunologically, pregnancy is something of a mystery. When a woman is pregnant, she is carrying a baby who is genetically non-identical to herself and yet she doesn't reject the baby as she would a kidney transplanted from that child. Surprisingly, a baby is not rejected despite the fact that there is only a wafer thin layer of cells between the mother and the child's blood and many proteins pass each way across this membrane of cells.

- The effect of the male hormone androgen: men suffer symptoms of allergic disease less often than women. However, it appears that the underlying allergic processes are still going on in the cells but due to the presence of the hormone androgen these do not give rise to symptoms. This is possibly one reason that explains why men have a shorter life expectancy than women.

- Women have more body fat than men: neotoxins are usually fat soluble and consequently stored in body fat. Women have a higher proportion of their bodyweight as subcutaneous fat, and consequently a greater reservoir of neotoxins to give them allergies.

- Women's livers are less active than men's. A woman's liver has less capacity to detoxify neotoxins, and so for the same intake of neotoxins, she is likely to suffer more symptoms. One worrying feature is the number of young women who are starting to drink and smoke considerably larger amounts than previously. This social change will increase the number of women suffering allergies to an even higher level.

THE SEVEN AGES OF WOMAN

As well as having double the rate of allergic disease, women also suffer from some allergic problems unique to females. These are listed below:

How can I beat Vaginal Thrush?

More than two out of five women in Britain gets vaginal thrush at some time in their lives. However, this is often a recurrent problem and is only the tip of an iceberg of hidden candida (yeast) infection of the bowel. The symptoms of vaginal thrush include an intense itching around the vulva and vagina, with or without a thick whitish discharge that looks like curdled milk. There may also be a burning sensation at the entrance to the vagina and sexual intercourse is painful. Although candida is blamed for a very wide variety of complaints, it is often itself just a sign of depressed immune and detoxification systems unable to cope.

Although candida gives obvious symptoms in the vagina, the real problem is in the large bowel, where the usual delicate balance of bacteria and candida has been disturbed in favour of candida. The local growth of candida releases poisonous toxins, which have a general toxic effect on the body, but also a specific effect on the womb, making it less responsive to normal levels of the hormone progesterone. The candida toxin also increases the likelihood and severity of the premenstrual syndrome (PMS see page 216).

Candida bowel infections and vaginal thrush are more likely to occur in women who have a poor general state of health with depressed immune and detoxification systems. It is also encouraged by a diet laden with yeast

Age	Common allergic problem or risk factor for allergy
0–9 yrs.	This is the single decade in which females have less allergic illness than males.
10–19 yrs.	Oral contraceptive (risk factor for many allergies); recurrent vaginal thrush; cystitis
20–29 yrs.	Infertility
30–39 yrs.	Pregnancy + PMS
40–49 yrs.	PMS Thyroid disease
50–59 yrs.	Menopause
60–69 yrs.	Osteoporosis

and sugars, by multiple pregnancies, and by drugs such as antibiotics, steroids and the oral contraceptive. The subject of candida infection is discussed in greater depth on page 181, and listed in Chapter 10 are the measures required to beat recurrent vaginal thrush without using drugs.

How can I beat cystitis?

Cystitis is the inflammation of the bladder and the urethra, which is the short tube that leads from the bladder to the outside. It affects at least half the women in Britain at sometime in their life. Women are much more vulnerable to cystitis than men because of the different anatomy which makes the bladder much more vulnerable to contamination by bacteria and candida. The symptoms of cystitis are:

- A very urgent and frequent desire to pass water although the amount of water passed is often very small and doesn't relieve the discomfort. Often the bladder still feels that it should be emptied;
- A burning sensation when passing water or a constant dull ache in the lower abdomen. On occasions, the pain can be so great that it is difficult to pass water;
- Blood in the urine.

There are several causes of cystitis.

Bacterial infection

This occurs because bacteria get into the bladder and multiply irritating the bladder wall causing inflammation. These bacteria usually rise from the bowel and this type of infection is encouraged by poor hygiene, sex or even wearing tight trousers. The bacterial infection causes dark or cloudy urine which may smell fishy and other symptoms suffered by the woman include a raised temperature, dull headache and flushes, as bacterial toxins enter the blood.

Non-bacterial infection

This is usually due to a candida infection around the entrance to the bladder and can be associated with vaginal thrush and itching around the anus (pruritis ani). Since this form of cystitis is caused by a yeast not a bacteria, an antibiotic will make the infection and symptoms worse.

Other irritants

Some food, e.g., curries, highly spiced foods and excessive amounts of alcohol, tea, coffee and fruit juices may give symptoms of cystitis in some women. In addition, local irritants such as deodorants, scented sprays, perfumed soaps and bubble baths, can cause this problem.

Bladder infections can usually be avoided or controlled by the following methods.

Hygiene

Keep the area around the vagina and anus clean and dry by daily washing. When washing and wiping, always work from front to back to avoid bacterial contamination of the bladder area. Avoid local irritants such as deodorants, scented sprays, perfumed soaps and bubble baths.

High fluid intake

Drink 3 to 4 pints preferably of bottled spring water a day and restrict intake of strong tea, coffee, alcohol and spicy foods. Empty the bladder every 3 to 4 hours as this flushes out infections.

Diet

Avoid foods rich in sugar, starch or yeast (see page 183). Also, suspect that your cystitis may be related to a particular food. By keeping a diet diary, you may be able to associated a particular food with your attacks. In order to prove this, try an exclusion diet and then

213

challenge yourself (see page 42).

Correct clothing

The bladder is most resistant to infection when this area is kept cool and dry by encouraging a free circulation of air. To do this wear cotton rather than synthetic fibre underwear, stockings rather than tights, and skirts or loose trousers.

Sex

Shower before sex, use plenty of lubrication, and pass urine within 15 minutes after sex.

Medication

Certain medications increase the risk of bacterial cystitis. These include steroids and the oral contraceptive pill. Candida/thrush is encouraged by the above two medications together with antibiotics.

If you find an attack of cystitis starting, increase your fluid intake by drinking a glass of water every 20 minutes and make your urine alkaline by taking a teaspoon of bicarbonate of soda in water every hour for the first three hours. You may find the homoeopathic medicine Cantharis 6 helpful, and you should take two tablets every three hours for the first 24 hours. The vitamin and mineral supplements that may help you beat cystitis include the B complex, Vitamin C, Vitamin E, magnesium, zinc, evening primrose oil, and acidophillus.

Does the oral contraceptive increase the risk of allergies?

The combined oral contraceptive ('the pill') contains both the female sex hormones oestrogen and progesterone. Consequently, it has a major effect on the metabolism of a woman's body. The oral contraceptive, particularly if taken for more than two years, increases the risk of allergies such as migraine,

food and chemical sensitivities, through depressing the immune and detoxification systems and thus causing vitamin and mineral deficiencies and encouraging overgrowth with candida. It also increases the risk of many female cancers, including cancer of the breast, cervix, ovary and womb. The best contraceptive alternatives to taking the pill are barrier methods such as the condom or natural family planning which, contrary to popular view, can be very successful when both the temperature and mucus method are used. For women who do not wish to stop taking the contraceptive pill, it is important to supplement the diet with Vitamin B complex, especially Vitamin B_6, Vitamin C, Vitamin E, magnesium, evening primrose oil, and especially zinc.

CAN ALLERGIES CAUSE INFERTILITY?

Any factor that affects general health also tends to reduce fertility. Allergic illnesses depress the immune and detoxification systems, which then reduce fertility. Curing these allergies and correcting vitamin and mineral deficiencies often also cures infertility.

A couple are said to be infertile if they fail to conceive after 2 years without contraception. About four out of five couples conceive within the first year of unprotected sex. Although the woman is usually blamed for infertility, in about one third of couples the problem is with the woman, in one third the problem is with the man and in the last third there is a joint problem.

Infertility is best treated by using 'pre-conceptual care' which is a method of taking ante-natal care one stage further, by looking at both partners before conception. At the moment of conception the man's contribution is just as important as the woman's. After that it is the woman's job to incubate the egg for 9 months and supply all the nutrients required by the growing baby. The benefit of pre-conceptual care is to reduce the number of miscarriages and still-births, and increase the number of normal healthy babies. Using these techniques, incidences of congenital problems like spina bifida can be reduced to almost zero. Unfortunately, the present system of ante-natal care starts much too late, since most congenital problems have occurred by 8 weeks after conception.

'Pre-conceptual care' uses the standard principles of Environmental Medicine, and looks at the whole body and lifestyle for any risk factors, by examining diet, occupation, housing, hobbies and social situation. Appropriate advice is then given to both the woman and the man to change their lifestyle to reduce their risk factors. This method works well for women who have already suffered miscarriages. The usual rate of miscarriage is one in four of all conceptions, however, miscarriages are much more likely to occur in women who have already suffered previous miscarriages.

What factors need to be considered to treat infertility?

- *Age*: this is of particular importance for women. The incidence of Down's syndrome and other problems increases after 37 years of age, and it may be wise to carry out an amniocentesis test at 16 weeks of pregnancy in order to rule out congenital abnormalities.
- *Occupation*: many jobs are associated with exposure to harmful chemicals, heavy metals, radiated energy and stress. All these may cause problems in a susceptible individual (see page 138).
- *General health*: chronic illness is quite common even in people of child-bearing age. Every attempt to cure or control any illness should be made before conception occurs.
- *Details of marriage/infertility*: it is important to know how long the couple have tried for a pregnancy, previous pregnancies, details of previous marriages and fertility.
- *Previous medical details*: relating to previous illnesses, operations especially abdominal operations, injuries, hospital treatments, dental treatments and medication taken. Infections are particularly important e.g. mumps in men and occasionally one or other partner may have had a venereal disease which will affect fertility. Symptomless low-level infections of the cervix sometimes prevent conception.
- *The woman's gynaecological and contraceptive details*: what age periods started, frequency of periods, type of menstrual flow, previous pregnancies and miscarriages, previous termination of pregnancy, lifelong contraceptive practices, use of oral contraceptive, use of IUD (coil), pelvic infection.
- *Health of family of both partners*: general health of all close family members together with number and health of offspring from each union is important, since many diseases, including infertility, are frequently inherited.
- *Cigarette intake*: there is now hard evidence that if either partner smokes there is an increased incidence of infertility, miscarriages and congenital malformations. In addition, pregnant mothers who smoke tend to produce underweight babies who are more liable to squints, hyperactivity and cot deaths.
- *Alcohol intake*: alcohol taken within 3 months of conception appears to encourage infertility, miscarriage and congenital abnormality. Sperm are very susceptible to damage by alcohol.

- *Drugs*: some drugs, both prescribed and otherwise, may cause damage to the health and fertility of one or other partners.
- *Allergic details*: health may be adversely affected by food allergies, chemical allergies to polluted air or water, illness from radiated energy or stress. If there are problems with any of these it may be necessary to do a food or chemical exclusion test. Chemicals in air, food or water may also affect the developing baby, e.g. pollution of tap water by female hormones arising from recycled sewage tends to feminize male babies.
- *Diet*: in order to estimate the daily intake of protein, carbohydrate, fat, salt, vitamins and minerals.

What tests need to be carried out to investigate infertility?

- Urine tests: to look for the presence of sugar, suggesting diabetes, and for protein, suggesting kidney or bladder problems.
- Blood tests: in order to establish general health, presence of anaemia or infections, liver or kidney problems, thyroid problems. Also to discover immunity or otherwise to rubella (German Measles) and if indicated, other infections such as toxoplasmosis and cytomegalovirus.
- Hair analysis: this is a technique which gives an accurate estimate of the body's levels of trace elements and toxic heavy metals. Analysing hair gives a very accurate assessment of the level of minerals *within* cells, whereas a blood test looks at the level of minerals in serum – the liquid between the blood cells rather than the cells themselves.
- Other tests: these may be carried out as required, or the result may already be available e.g. recent cervical smear, semen analysis, temperature chart using fertility thermometer.

How soon after pre-conceptual care should we plan a pregnancy?

After you have made appropriate changes to diet, occupation, housing, hobbies and social situation, stopped smoking, drinking alcohol and started taking vitamin and mineral supplements, your level of fertility is likely to improve. However, it is important to be in this state for 6 months before conception. This is because for the three months prior to conception, both the egg and the sperm are maturing and are especially vulnerable to damage. Damage prior to this period is of less importance. Thus in the six month plan, the first three months are to put both male and female into peak health, so that they can produce the highest quality egg and sperm in the second three month period. A healthy egg and healthy sperm will produce a healthy baby.

What vitamin and mineral supplements does the average person need prior to conception?

The typical vitamins and minerals needed pre-conceptually by the average person who does not have any specific deficiency are vitamin A, vitamin B complex, vitamin C, vitamin E, magnesium, zinc and evening primrose oil.

WHAT IS THE PREMENSTRUAL SYNDROME (PMS)?

This is a very common cyclical problem that affects three out of four women seriously enough to seek a remedy, and is a major disruption to the life of one woman in four. It commonly occurs between the ages of 25 to 40, and usually gets worse closer to the menopause.

Up to 150 different symptoms have been attributed to PMS, but the classic ones are:

Breast tenderness;

Fluid retention, bloating and weight gain;

Irritability, aggression and mood swings;

Depression and tiredness;

Poor co-ordination and clumsiness;

Concentration and memory problems;

Addiction to foods, with increased appetite and thirst.

Other symptoms: PMS can affect all systems of the body, and other symptoms include headaches and migraine, muscular aches and backache, cystitis, dizziness, fainting, hot sweats, cold flushes, nausea and vomiting, asthma, acne and skin eruptions, anxiety and restlessness, tension, frequent accidents, indecision, insomnia and withdrawal from society.

The diagnosis of PMS can be made only if symptoms are related to the menstrual cycle. The symptoms need to be present in the 10–15 days before menstruation, but need to be absent for about 7 days after menstruation. In order to confirm the diagnosis, you should fill in a menstrual diary, listed below, marking the squares with the following letters, for symptoms: B – Breast tenderness, F – Fluid retention, I – Irritability, D – Depression, P – Poor co-ordination, C – Concentration problems, A – Addiction to foods, M – Menstruation.

The premenstrual syndrome occurs because of fluctuations in the hormones oestrogen and progesterone during the menstrual cycle as shown in Figure 15.1. These hormones affect the permeability of the gut and the admission of undigested foods into the body.

Which factors make PMS worse?

There are many factors that make PMS worse, but they are related to high levels of neotoxins. Factors that depress the immune and detoxification systems:

● Fast food diet, full of sugar, additives, animal fats and saturated fats;

Table 15.1 **Menstrual Diary**

Days of month:

	1	2	3	4	5	6	7	8	9	10	11	12	13	14	15	16	17	18	19	20	21	22	23	24	25	26	27	28	29	30	31
Month																															
Month																															
Month																															

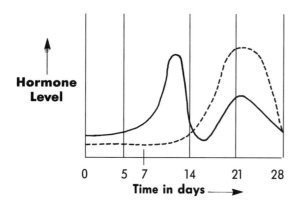

Key
Oestrogen = ——————
Progesterone = - - - - - - -

Figure 15.1 **Hormone level fluctuation during menstrual cycle**

- Alcohol and tobacco;
- Candida overgrowth;
- Drugs, including steroids, antibiotics, and the oral contraceptive pill which may causes overgrowth of candida;
- A stressful lifestyle at home, or work;
- Lack of exercise;
- Pregnancy;
- After surgery and anaesthetics.

What measures will make PMS better?

PMS can be considerably helped by the following measures:

- Reduction of intake of sugar and salt, junk food, additives, tea, coffee, chocolate, alcohol and cigarettes, all of which depress the immune and detoxification systems;
- Losing weight, reduction in intake of animal fats;
- Reduction in stress level;
- Regular exercise;

- Eating organic foods, and drinking bottled spring water, and breathing clean air;
- Taking the following vitamin and mineral supplements; vitamin B complex, especially vitamin B_6, vitamin C, vitamin E, magnesium, zinc and evening primrose oil and acidophillus.

CAN MYXOEDEMA BE DUE TO ALLERGIES?

Some forms of myxoedema occur after the immune system becomes confused and starts producing antibodies to the thyroid gland. This autoimmune process is much commoner in women, and is also encouraged by candida toxins. By correcting food allergies, chemical sensitivities and reducing the mass candida in the gut, it is possible to successfully treat some cases of myxoedema.

DOES PREGNANCY INCREASE THE RISK OF ALLERGY?

Pregnancy, especially repeated pregnancy, is a major direct and indirect cause of allergies and also many other non-allergic diseases. As a general rule, the greater the number of pregnancies the woman has, the shorter her life expectancy and the greater her risk of allergy. The allergies don't start until after pregnancy and existing ones may even get better at this time due to the high level of circulating hormones. However, problems frequently begin soon after the baby is born. The reasons pregnancy may exacerbate or act as a trigger factor for allergies include:

- High hormone levels and hormone fluctuations (especially at the beginning and end of the pregnancy). These hormone levels induce a greater than usual permeability in the gut which then allows more undigested foods into the bloodstream to challenge the immune and detoxification systems.

- During pregnancy the immune and detoxification systems are working overtime because of the large amount of foreign proteins and waste products arising from the baby which enter the mother's circulation via the placenta for processing. Consequently, there is far less spare capacity than usual to deal with any extra challenge to the immune and detoxification systems.
- Nutritional deficiencies are more likely to occur during pregnancy when the growing baby takes large amounts of proteins, vitamins and minerals from the mother at a faster rate than she can replace them with an unsupplemented diet. In the past it was a rule of thumb that a woman would lose one tooth for each child born because of the calcium taken from her by the unborn baby.
- High levels of hormones and a raised blood sugar level make a candida overgrowth of the bowel more common. Candida is quite likely to cause problems after the second or following pregnancies and the raised level of candida then acts as a further depressive influence on the immune and detoxification systems.
- Pregnancy is often a time of immense mental stress which, like any other neotoxin, has a depressive effect on the immune and detoxification systems. The stress that arises from life-event changes such as changing work pattern, suffering reduction of income, possibly moving house and living a totally different lifestyle looking after a highly dependent infant that requires 24 hour care. This is on top of the effort of growing a baby for 9 months and a painful labour.

HOW CAN ENVIRONMENTAL MEDICINE HELP WITH THE MENOPAUSE?

The menopause is a time in a woman's life when the ovaries stop producing the hormone oestrogen and the periods cease. It usually happens between the ages of 45 and 55 years, at present it affects 10 million women in Britain. Women differ from almost all other animals which remain fertile until their death, but the average woman will live a third of her life after she has stopped ovulating. Historically, it is a new phenomenon for women to live much of their life in the menopause. As recently as 1900 the average life expectancy of women was only 51 years, which is the average age of the start of the menopause.

The typical symptoms of the menopause are:

- **Autonomic problems:** flushes, sweats, dizziness, palpitations and migraine headaches;
- **Psychological problems:** irritability, depression, mood swings, anxiety, agoraphobia, panic attacks, loss in concentration and memory, tired all the time, insomnia;
- **Musculoskeletal problems:** joint and muscular pains, osteoporosis;
- **Biochemical changes:** rise in sodium level, weight gain, rise in blood cholesterol;
- **Sexual changes:** shrinkage of breasts, vaginal dryness, painful intercourse, loss of libido, bladder symptoms, thinning of skin, dry hair.

You will recognize many of the above symptoms as they may be caused by allergies, although it is important for your doctor to first rule out other medical problems such as anaemia, thyroid disease, and the side-effects of drugs. In many cases the allergic symptoms can be removed, or at least controlled, by using the techniques of Environmental Medicine. Remedies which have been found to assist menopausal symptoms include:

- Reducing your total load of neotoxins, and taking clean air, clean food and clean water. Stopping or reducing tobacco, alcohol, coffee and sugar consumption to the minimum;

- Regular vigorous exercise;

- Mineral and vitamin supplements including Vitamin A, Vitamin B complex and folic acid, Vitamin C, Vitamin D, Vitamin E, calcium, magnesium, zinc, fish oils and evening primrose oil.

CHAPTER SIXTEEN

CANCER

The dramatic rise in the incidence of cancer is one of the major penalties that we pay for our modern way of living. Even as little as one hundred years ago, a cancer death was the exception, whereas now one in three of the population dies from cancer. The reason for this rapid rise in cancer is the widespread pollution of air, food and water. Consequently, the techniques of Environmental Medicine are very powerful tools in the treatment of cancer, but even more importantly, Environmental Medicine is the key to avoiding cancer.

WHAT IS THE UNDERLYING PROCESS IN CANCER?

Cancer is often presented as a single-system disease, e.g. cancer of the lung, whereas in fact in almost all cases, it is a multi-system disease affecting all the major organs. This is in common with other degenerative diseases such as arthritis, heart disease and mental illness, which are also multi-system diseases. Cancer especially affects the immune system, in the blood and the white cells, and the detoxification system in the liver. The other common misconception is that cancer suddenly just happens. In fact it occurs at the end of a progression from health through possibly an allergic illness to a pre-cancer state and then finally to cancer (see Table 16.1). This pre-

cancer state persists for some time and if the factors causing it are not removed, then a cancer proper starts to grow.

Although cancer sometimes runs in families, it is estimated that 75 per cent of cancers are related to environmental factors (neotoxins). The common neotoxins causing pre-cancer state are:

- The wrong diet (e.g., food additives, high salt and fat, low fibre);
- Viruses (e.g., papilloma virus);
- Chemical carcinogens (e.g., drugs, such as the oral contraceptive, smoking, asbestos, dyes, soot, vinyl chloride, arsenic, chromium and nickel);
- Radiation (e.g., UV light, X-rays and powerful, non-ionizing radiation);
- Stress (e.g., road accident).

Over years, the total load of neotoxins causes a slow poisoning of the liver's ability to detoxify chemicals and also reactivate the oxidizing enzymes essential for healthy metabolism. It also depresses the immune system and this loses its ability to launch the inflammatory response which identifies and then destroys cancer cells. The reason that pre-cancer cells occur is because normal metabolism no longer takes place and the liver, which is the biggest single organ in the body, stops working properly. During the pre-cancer state,

Table 16.1 **Development of Cancer**

Youth/Middle Age			Middle/Old Age
Health + neotoxins →	Allergy + neotoxins →	Precancer state + neotoxins →	Cancer
Normal immune and detoxification systems.	Immune and detoxification systems are not functioning properly.	Loss of normal inflammatory response. Damage to liver and detoxification system. Precancer cells become more negative and conduct electricity better than normal cells. Drop in potassium level within cells affects hormones, vitamins and enzymes.	More damage to liver which becomes unable to reactivate bodies oxidizing enzymes. Cancer cells regress to resemble embryonic cells with high sodium and low potassium content. Energy is obtained using anaerobic metabolism which produces lactic acid which accelerates cell growth. Cell shape and function becomes very primitive.

allergic symptoms like migraine often disappear and cells, especially liver cells, lose the mineral potassium (K) and allow the entry of the mineral sodium (Na). The potassium/sodium ratio in the cell is very important, because this ratio, together with the acidity (pH), governs the activity of a wide variety of hormones, vitamins and enzymes.

Pre-cancer cells do not act like normal cells and their reduced potassium causes them to be more electronegative than the normal cell with an increased electrical conductivity. After a variable period in the pre-cancer state, a trigger factor (e.g., a virus infection or massive exposure to chemicals, shock, or accident) may precipitate cancer growth.

Cancer cells resemble primitive embryonic cells; they change their shape from the usual dimensions, change their metabolism, and the nucleus, when viewed under the microscope, takes up a stain much more avidly than before. The potassium level within the cell drops and the sodium level rises, and energy is produced by the inefficient method of anaerobic metabolism which converts glucose to lactic acid which further stimulates cell growth. This tumour growth causes the liver to swell and it is no longer able to reactivate essential oxidizing enzymes which are necessary to detoxify substances usually circulating in the blood. The depressive effect of a growing cancer can be shown by the fact that when that cancer is surgically removed, liver function tests improve.

WHAT DECIDES WHICH TYPE OF CANCER DEVELOPS?

This is another example of the 'Weak Link Theory'. Although any cancer *could* occur at any time in life, age and sex are the predictive factors which decide the organ most likely to

Age	Male	Female
0–9 yrs	Leukaemias Kidney, Central Nervous System and Congenital tumours	Leukaemias Kidney, Central Nervous System and Congenital tumours
10–19yrs	Lymphoma and Bone Sarcoma (rare)	Lymphoma and Bone Sarcoma (rare)
20–29yrs	Testicular tumours	Melanoma Skin tumour (rare)
30–39yrs	Testicular tumours	Breast tumour (rare)
40–49yrs	Stomach Pancreas Bladder tumours	Breast Stomach Pancreas tumours
50–59yrs	Lung Stomach Colon Prostate Pancreas Bladder tumours	Breast, Cervix Stomach Colon Lung Pancreas Oesophagus Cervix tumours
60 yrs +	Lung Colon Leukaemias Prostate Skin, Pancreas Bladder Oesophagus tumours	Colon Breast Lung Leukaemias Skin, Pancreas Ovary Uterus tumours

Table 16.2 **Peak incidence of cancer by organ**

be affected. Cancers are most common among people over 60 years, although there is a moderately high incidence of cancers in the very young (0–2 years). As a general rule, the earlier in life a cancer starts growing the more rapid its increase in size and likelihood of spreading. In contrast, cancers starting after 60 years of age are often slow-growing. Even without treatment of these tumours, death may occur apparently for a different reason, e.g., a heart attack. However, it must be remembered that this disease probably develops because of the same disturbed metabolism that causes the cancer growth.

WHY IS THERE SUCH AN ENORMOUS WORLDWIDE VARIATION IN THE INCIDENCE OF CANCER?

There is an enormous variation in the incidence of cancer in different countries. This is directly related to the level of pollution of air, food and water. Cancer levels are high in polluted industrialized countries in which the diet is highly processed and full of additives, e.g., western Europe, but cancer is almost unknown amongst the Hunza tribe, who live in a completely unpolluted site on the slopes of the Himalayas, eating only organic, unprocessed foods and not coming into contact with varied sources of chemicals.

Incidence of cancer is also influenced by genetic and racial characteristics, e.g., Central Africans have a very high incidence of liver tumours. However, this incidence of cancer is highly dependent on their diet and when the type of food they eat is changed the incidence of cancer drops dramatically. Residents of Southern Italy and Greece have a low cancer rate, which is probably related to their high intake of garlic.

WHAT IS THE RISK OF AN INDIVIDUAL CELL BECOMING CANCEROUS?

The risk of any individual cell becoming cancerous is very, very low, but when you consider that there are 10^{12} cells (i.e., a million million cells) in the human body, it requires only one cell in a million to become cancerous each day to produce a million cancer cells daily. Fortunately, this does not happen, because when the metabolism is healthy very few cells become pre-cancerous and the immune system is able to spot such cells.

It is particularly important that the body is able to detect cancer cells at a very early stage before they have time to divide again and again, and form a large ball of tumour cells. Such large tumour masses are much more difficult to destroy, because the outer cells prevent the antibodies and white cells of the immune system from getting to the growing centre, whereas when the mass is very small the inner cells have relatively little protection.

This concept of the ratio of area/volume of cancer cell mass also explains why skin cancers tend to grow relatively easily when the immune system is depressed a little. When such tumours grow on the surface they have a 180° that is free from attack by the immune system. However, it is noticeable that such skin tumours, especially melanomas, are very responsive to methods that boost the immune system and normalize metabolism.

WHAT SYMPTOMS AND SIGNS MIGHT SUGGEST CANCER?

The secret of successful cancer management is early diagnosis. There are now screening programmes set up for early diagnosis of many tumours, especially for high risk groups, e.g., smokers. Cancer of the cervix is found by a cervical smear. Breast cancer is found by an X-ray mammography. Lung cancer is found by routine chest X-ray. Cancer of the colon can be found by looking for blood in the motions and using a sigmoidoscope to view the colon directly. Testicular cancer is found by self-examination. Cancer of the ovary can be found by looking for the presence of a marker in the blood.

The signs which should make you suspect cancer include unexpected loss of blood from any orifice, unexplained pain or soreness, persistent hoarseness of voice, or any lump that changes in size, colour or outline. If you notice any of these changes, seek medical advice without delay.

HOW DOES THE WRONG DIET CAUSE CANCER?

The problem is that 'sick food makes sick people'. Approximately 40 per cent of cancers in men are associated with dietary errors. Modern food cultivation methods force food to grow too quickly in soil that has been exhausted through being over-worked and not allowed to stand fallow between growing periods. Instead of using manure to make up

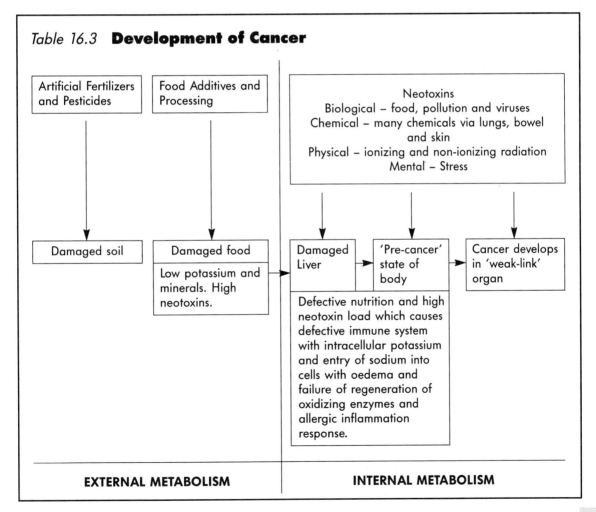

Table 16.3 **Development of Cancer**

for the nitrogen and minerals taken out, artificial fertilizers are added. The result is food which is nutritionally inferior due to reduced levels of vitamins and minerals. Spraying of the food with pesticides followed by modern processing methods, e.g. incorporation of food additives, creates a food which further precipitates allergic symptoms or else slowly poisons the immune and detoxification systems. In this way, problems with the 'external metabolism' give rise to problems with the 'internal metabolism'. This is the reason why it is so important not to pollute our environment because we are paid back with ill health. As a general rule, what is good for the environment is also good for the individual.

HOW CAN THE CORRECT DIET BE USED TO AVOID CANCER?

The external metabolism can be made healthy by growing food organically, i.e., in a soil that doesn't have any artificial fertilizers, pesticides or chemicals applied to it. The food is then harvested, stored and transported without use of pesticides or chemicals and will contain high levels of vitamins and minerals with no neotoxins and is consequently very nourishing. If water and air intake are also free of neotoxins, then the internal metabolism will work well and the fully functioning detoxification and immune system will make the body very cancer resistant (see Table 16.4).

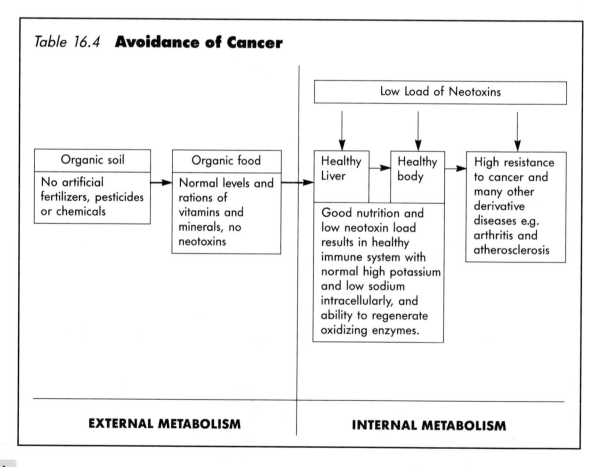

Table 16.4 **Avoidance of Cancer**

EXTERNAL METABOLISM | INTERNAL METABOLISM

WHAT EFFECT DO STRESS AND UNHAPPINESS HAVE ON CANCER GROWTH?

Mental stress, including bereavement, shock, unhappiness or frustration all increase the likelihood of cancer growth because they generate dangerous free radicals which can overwhelm the immune and detoxification systems. In many ways, a bad thought is as dangerous as a bad chemical. Conversely, feeling happy, loved, fulfilled and successful is protective, since these thoughts generate natural opiates called endorphins which assist the immune and detoxification systems in fighting cancer. This explains the success of positive visualization as a useful technique in beating cancer.

WHAT OTHER LIFE CHANGES CAN I MAKE TO AVOID CANCER?

The most important life-change that smokers can make to reduce their risk of cancer is to stop smoking. This could save almost four out of five lung and larynx cancer deaths under the age of 65, and about a quarter of the deaths from cancer of the pancreas, bladder and cervix. Occupational exposure is an important factor for many cancers, especially cancer of the lung and bladder and the factors implicated are asbestos and dyes respectively. Alcohol intake is an important risk factor for cancer of the mouth and larynx. Ultra-violet light (and ionizing radiation) is an important risk factor for skin cancer and may come from bright sunlight and sunbeds. Non-ionizing radiation from high voltage power lines and radio and microwave transmitters may increase the likelihood of leukaemias.

HOW SHOULD CANCER BE TREATED?

Conventional medicine uses the following techniques with a varying degree of success:

Surgery
Chemotherapy
Radiotherapy
Hormone Therapy
Immunotherapy

Apart from immunotherapy, these treatments do not assist the immune and detoxification systems to regenerate themselves. Furthermore, radiotherapy and especially chemotherapy give these two systems an enormous extra load of neotoxins to process. Cancer cells are unable to change back to normal cells and so to get rid of cancer these cells have to be killed by the immune system. To do this, the body must be able to mount an inflammatory response causing redness and local swelling at the site of the tumour followed a day or two later by a reduction in the swelling and digestion of the cancer cells by white cells. Then there is growth of capilliaries and healing. The inflammatory process will not start until the immune and detoxification systems have been boosted by reducing the total load of neotoxins and clearing vitamin and mineral deficiencies.

The treatment of cancer based on principles of Environmental Medicine has the following elements:

● Reducing the total load of neotoxins by taking clean food, clean air, and clean water. The food needs to be organic, the water bottled spring water and the air pollution free. Foods such as animal fats, animal proteins, and salt encourage the growth of cancer and should be avoided. Foods that protect against cancer are fresh organic fruit and vegetables and their juices, unprocessed carbohydrates, and freshly pressed fruit juices which contain highly active enzymes.

- If there is any particularly dangerous neotoxin in the environment then this should be completely avoided.
- Use sleep, rest, exercise, vitamin and mineral supplements to return to health. The vitamins required include high doses of Vitamin A, B complex, folic acid, Vitamin C, Vitamin E, potassium, calcium, magnesium, selenium, zinc, fish oils and evening primrose oil.

CHAPTER SEVENTEEN

CONCLUSIONS

This chapter is deliberately brief so as not to dilute its message.

- In the latter part of the twentieth century, pollution of air, food and water is increasingly common and responsible for the explosion in allergic disease.
- The natural state of the body is health, and an allergic symptom or disease indicates a mistake in your lifestyle (i.e. diet, occupation, housing, hobbies or social situation).
- In order to get well, you must make an active decision to change your lifestyle. To do this successfully you must plan to start your new lifestyle with adequate resources.
- The typical approach of conventional medicine to allergic disease is to use powerful drugs to suppress symptoms and treat single organs. This method, unfortunately, has limited success. Environmental Medicine has a far greater success by treating the whole body. This is done by removing sources of neotoxins and correcting deficiencies of vitamins and minerals which then encourage the immune and detoxification systems to work properly.
- The three rules of Environmental Medicine treatment are:
  1. *Reduce your total load of neotoxins* by taking clean air, clean food and clean water.
  2. *Reduce particularly the neotoxin to which you are especially sensitive.*
  3. *Use sleep, rest, exercise, vitamins, minerals and other supplements to help yourself back to complete health.*

APPENDIX

FOOD FAMILIES

Food families are very useful ways of classifying foods. All members of a single food family are recognized by the body as being of similar origin. Someone who is allergic to one food is more likely to be allergic to other members of the same food family. Food families are of particular importance when designing exclusion and rotary diets. As a general rule, the further away from your home that a food grows, the less likely you are to be allergic to it. For example, rice grows in Asia, and rice allergy is rare in people who have lived in England all their life.

FOOD FAMILIES (PLANTS)

Banana family	– banana
Beech family	– chestnut
Borage family	– borage, comfrey
Buckwheat family	– buckwheat, rhubarb
Cactus family	– prickly pear
Carrot family	– carrot, celery, chervil, coriander, cumin, dill, fennel, parsley, parsnip
Cashew family	– cashew nuts, mango, pistachio
Citrus family	– grapefruit, kumquat, lemon, lime, orange, satsuma, tangerine
Composite family	– artichoke, chamomile, chicory, dandelion, endive, globe lettuce, pyrethrum, safflower oil, sunflower (all forms), tarragon
Dillenia family	– kiwi fruit (chinese gooseberry)
Fungi	– alcohol, bakers yeast, mushrooms, vinegar, certain vitamins (see page 183 for yeast-free diet)
Ginger family	– cardomom, ginger, tumeric
Goosefoot family	– beet, spinach, sugar beet
Gourd family	– cantelope, courgettes, cucumber, gherkin, marrow, pumpkin, (water) melon
Grape family	– grape, brandy, champagne, cream of tartar, raisin, sultanas, all wines, wine vinegar
Grass (western)	– barley, corn (all forms), malt, maltose, oats, popcorn, sugar cane
Grass (eastern)	– bamboo shoots, millet, sorghum, rice
Heath family	– blueberry, cranberry, huckleberry

Honeysuckle family	– elderberry
Laurel family	– avocado, bayleaf, cinnamon
Legumes (also called pulses)	– beans, (blackeyed, fava, lima, mung, navy, string), carob, chickpea, gum acacia and tragacanth, lentil, liquorice, pea, peanut, senna, soy bean, soya (all forms), tamarind
Lily family	– Aloe vera, asparagus, chives, garlic, leek, onion, shallot
Maple family	– maple syrup
Mint family	– basil, lavender, lemon balm, marjoram, oregano, peppermint, rosemary, sage, spearmint, thyme
Morning Glory family	– sweet potato
Mulberry family	– breadfruit, fig, hop, mulberry
Mustard family	– broccoli, Brussels sprouts, cabbage, cauliflower, chinese cabbage, horseradish, cale, mustard seed, radish, rape, swede, turnip, watercress
Myrtle family	– cloves, eucalyptus, guava
Nutmeg family	– nutmeg, mace
Olive family	– olive and olive oil
Orchid family	– vanilla
Palm family	– coconut, date, sago
Papaya family	– papaya
Passion Flower family	– passion fruit
Pedalium family	– sesame seed, tahini
Pepper family	– peppercorn, black pepper, white pepper
Pineapple family	– pineapple
Pomegranate family	– pomegrante, grenadine
Potato family	– pepper (Capsicum), cayenne, chili, paprika, potato, tobacco, tomato
Rose family	–
1). pomes	– apple, cider, cider vinegar, pectin, crabapple, pear, quince, rosehip
2). stone fruits	– almond, apricot, cherry, nectarine, peach, plum, prune, sloe
3). berries	– blackberry, loganberry, raspberry, strawberry
Sapodilla family	– chewing gum
Sapucaya family	– brazil nut, paradise nut
Saxifrage family	– blackcurrant, currants, gooseberry, recurrants, whitecurrants
Soapberry family	– lychee
Spurge family	– cassava, tapioca, castor bean
Sterculia family	– chocolate, cocoa, cola nut
Tea	– tea
Walnut family	– English walnut, hickory nut, pecan
Yam family	– Chinese Potato (Yam)

The following is a list of plants in which each case is the only member of a food family that is *commonly* eaten. Cross-sensitivity (reactivity with another member of the same family) is unlikely to occur with these foods: avocado, banana, black pepper, brazil nut, chestnut, elderberry, fig, ginseng, hazelnut, juniper, kiwi fruit, lychee, maple, olive, pineapple, sweet potato, sesame (tahini), tapioca, vanilla (natural), yam.

FOOD FAMILIES (ANIMALS)

Mammals

The Bovine family

Beef – meat, rennet or rennin, sausage casings, suet

Milk – milk, butter, cheese, ice cream, lactose, yoghurt, why and caesin (see page 51 for milk-free diet)

Goat – goats' milk, goats' cheese, goats' ice cream

Sheep – lamb and mutton, ewes' milk, ewes' cheese

Other Mammal Food Families

Deer family – caribou, deer, elk, moose, reindeer
Hare family – hare and rabbit
Horse family – horse
Swine family – bacon, ham, lard, pork, sausage

Bird Food Families

Duck family – duck and duck eggs, goose and goose eggs
Dove family – dove, pigeon
Grouse family – grouse and partridge
Pheasant family – chicken and chicken eggs, pea fowl, pheasant, quail
Turkey family – turkey and turkey eggs

Fish Food Families

Codfish – cod, coley, haddock, hake
Flatfish – dab, flounder, halibut, plaice, sole
Herring – herring, pilchard, sardine
Mackerel – mackerel, skipjack, tuna
Salmon – salmon, trout
Molluscs – clam, mussel, oyster, scallop, snail, squib
Crustacean (Shellfish) – crab, crayfish, lobster, prawn, shrimp

The following animals are the only members of their food family that are *commonly* eaten. Allergy is unlikely to occur due to cross-activity without another member of the same food family: anchovy, deer, rabbit, sturgeon, turkey, whitefish.

Table A.1 **Normal height and weight for boys**

The following table gives the range of height and weight for boys between birth and 18 years of age. If your child is not within the limits for height or weight then he should be seen by your doctor to find out the cause of this abnormality. Once other causes have been ruled out, testing for allergy can be started.

NOTE: 1 stone (st) = 14 pounds (lb).

BOYS

Age	Height range (ft ins)	Weight range (st lbs)
Birth		5.5lb – 9.6lb
3 months	1'8" – 2'1"	9.6lb – 15.9lb
6 months	2'0" – 2'3"	13.6lb – 1st 5lb

	BOYS	
Age	Height range (ft ins)	Weight range (st lbs)
9 months	2'1" – 2'5"	1st 2lb – 1st 8lb
12 months	2'3" – 2'6"	1st 3lb – 2st 0lb
18 months	2'4" – 2'8"	1st 4lb – 2st 3lb
2 years	2'6" – 3'0"	1st 8lb – 2st 4lb
3 years	2'8" – 3'3"	1st 9lb – 2st 8lb
4 years	3'0" – 3'6"	2st 0lb – 3st 3lb
5 years	3'2" – 3'8"	2st 2lb – 3st 6lb
6 years	3'4" – 4'0"	2st 5lb – 4st 2lb
7 years	3'6" – 4'2"	2st 6lb – 4st 7lb
8 years	3'7" – 4'5"	2st 9lb – 5st 3lb
9 years	3'9" – 4'7"	3st 3lb – 6st 1lb
10 years	4'1" – 4'8"	3st 6lb – 6st 9lb
11 years	4'2" – 5'0"	3st 9lb – 7st 8lb
12 years	4'3" – 5'2"	4st 2lb – 9st 1lb
13 years	4'5" – 5'5"	4st 7lb – 10st 0lb
14 years	4'7" – 5'7"	5st 1lb – 11st 1lb
15 years	4'9" – 5'9"	6st 1lb – 11st 9lb
16 years	5'1" – 6'0"	7st 2lb – 12st 4lb
17 years	5'3" – 6'1"	7st 7lb – 12st 6lb
18 years	5'3" – 6'1"	7st 9lb – 12st 9lb

Table A.2 **Normal height and weight for girls**

The following table gives the range of height and weight for girls between birth and 18 years of age. If your child is not within the limits for height or weight then she should be seen by your doctor to find out the cause of this abnormality. Once other causes have been ruled out, testing for allergy can be started.

NOTE: 1 stone (st) = 14 pounds (lb).

GIRLS

Age	Height range (ft ins)	Weight range (st lbs)
Birth		5.5lb – 9.6lb
3 months	1'8" – 2'0"	9.2lb – 15.4lb
6 months	2'0" – 2'3"	13.6lb – 1st 5lb
9 months	2'1" – 2'4"	1st 1lb – 1st 7lb
12 months	2'2" – 2'5"	1st 2lb – 1st 9lb
18 months	2'4" – 2'8"	1st 3lb – 2st 1lb
2 years	2'6" – 3'0"	1st 5lb – 2st 3lb
3 years	2'8" – 3'3"	1st 7lb – 2st 7lb
4 years	3'0" – 3'6"	2st 0lb – 3st 1lb
5 years	3'2" – 3'8"	2st 3lb – 3st 6lb
6 years	3'4" – 4'0"	2st 5lb – 4st 2lb
7 years	3'6" – 4'2"	2st 9lb – 4st 7lb
8 years	3'8" – 4'4"	2st 9lb – 5st 5lb
9 years	3'9" – 4'7"	3st 3lb – 6st 2lb
10 years	4'1" – 4'8"	3st 6lb – 7st 5lb
11 years	4'2" – 5'0"	3st 9lb – 8st 8lb
12 years	4'4" – 5'4"	4st 4lb – 10st 0lb
13 years	4'6" – 5'5"	5st 2lb – 11st 0lb
14 years	4'8" – 5'6"	5st 8lb – 11st 4lb
15 years	4'9" – 5'7"	6st 6lb – 11st 6lb
16 years	5'0" – 5'7"	7st 0lb – 11st 8lb
17 years		7st 2lb – 11st 7lb
18 years		7st 2lb – 11st 7lb

Table A.3 **Normal height and weight for adult males**
Maximum desirable weight for men aged 25 plus
NOTE: 1 stone (st) = 14 pounds (lb)

Height without shoes		BODY FRAME					
		Small		Medium		Large	
ft in	m	st lbs	kg	st lbs	kg	st lbs	kg
5 3	1.60	8 9	55	9 7	60	10 4	65
5 4	1.63	9 0	57	9 10	62	10 8	67

Height without shoes		BODY FRAME					
		Small		Medium		Large	
5 5	1.65	9 3	59	9 13	63	10 12	69
5 6	1.68	9 7	60	10 3	65	11 2	71
5 7	1.70	9 11	62	10 7	67	11 7	73
5 8	1.73	10 1	64	10 12	69	11 12	75
5 9	1.75	10 5	66	11 2	71	12 1	77
5 10	1.78	10 10	68	11 6	73	12 6	79
5 11	1.80	11 0	70	11 11	75	12 11	81
6 0	1.83	11 4	72	12 2	77	13 2	84
6 1	1.85	11 8	74	12 7	80	13 7	86
6 2	1.88	11 13	76	12 12	82	13 12	88

Instructions: Weigh yourself in indoor clothes wearing shoes.
Subtract 7 pounds (3.2 kilos) if naked.

Table A.4 **Normal height and weight for adult females**

Maximum desirable weight for women aged 25 plus
NOTE: 1 stone (st) = 14 pounds (lb)

Height without shoes		BODY FRAME					
		Small		Medium		Large	
ft in	m	st lbs	kg	st lbs	kg	st lbs	kg
4 11	1.50	7 3	46	7 12	50	8 10	55
5 0	1.52	7 6	47	8 1	51	8 13	57
5 1	1.55	7 9	49	8 4	53	9 2	58
5 2	1.57	7 12	50	8 7	54	9 5	60
5 3	1.60	8 1	51	8 10	55	9 8	61
5 4	1.63	8 4	53	9 0	57	9 12	63
5 5	1.65	8 7	54	9 4	59	10 2	65
5 6	1.68	8 11	56	9 9	61	10 6	66
5 7	1.70	9 0	58	9 13	63	10 10	68
5 8	1.73	9 5	60	10 3	65	11 0	70
5 9	1.75	9 9	61	10 7	67	11 4	72
5 10	1.78	10 0	64	10 11	69	11 9	74

Instructions: Weigh yourself in indoor clothes wearing shoes.
Subtract 5 pounds (2.25 kilos) if you are naked.

GLOSSARY

Adaption: The process in which the body gets used to a neotoxin and is able to break it down by activation enzymes.

Allergen: A substance that causes an allergy.

Allergy: There are many definitions for this work. Von Pirquet used it to describe a state of altered reactivity which occurred after exposure to a specific environmental factor. Some doctors use a very narrow definition of allergy which they say occurs only when there is an antigen/antibody reaction in the blood. An allergy may occur at any exposure after the first.

Anaphylaxis: A severe, rapidly occurring allergic reaction caused by the release of histamines from mast cells. It can cause collapse, low blood pressure and sometimes even death.

Antibody: This is a protein (immunoglobulin) produced by white cells in order to protect the body against foreign (non-self) substances.

Antigen: A substance, usually a protein, that provokes antibody production and allergic response.

Antihistamine: A drug that blocks the effect of histamine (q.v.).

Antioxidant: A chemical or vitamin which stops molecular oxygen from working as an unwanted oxidizing agent or free radical. The commonest antioxidants in common use are Vitamin C, Vitamin E, selenium and superoxide dismutase (SOD).

Atopy: A hereditary tendency to allergic diseases such as asthma, eczema, hayfever.

Bioaccumulation: The build up of a chemical in the body. This is usually a lipid soluble chemical building up in the fat.

Bipolarity: This is a basic phenomenon of allergy in which a single neotoxin at first stimulates, followed by a depressant effect with withdrawal symptoms due to a failure of the adapted enzyme system to cope.

Carcinogen: A substance or factor that encourages the growth of a cancer.

Candida: A yeast also known as monila

or thrush, which is a fungus or mould.

Catalyst: A substance which is able to increase the rate of a chemical reaction. The catalyst need be present only in a very small amount and is not used up in the chemical reaction.

Coherent waves: These are waves of the same frequency which are moving in phase (in step).

Dander: Skin of an animal which, separate from the animal hair, may cause an allergic reaction.

Electric field: This is produced by an electric charge at rest, or alternatively, may be induced by a magnetic field. It is measured in volts per meter.

Electromagnetic field (EMF): This is a combined electric and magnetic field.

Enzyme: A protein produced by a cell which acts as a biological catalyst.

Free radicals: Free radicals are the mechanism by which neotoxins produce allergies. They are very short-lived molecules and are necessary for the cell to release energy. However, excess free radicals overwhelm the cells' ability to quench them, are highly dangerous and produce tissue damage by punching holes in cell membranes. They can be removed by Vitamin C, Vitamin E, selenium and superoxide dismutase.

Frequency: Frequency is the number of complete oscillations per second of a wave. It is measured in cycles per second (Hertz). Frequency is inversely proportional to wavelength.

Histamine: A protein released by mast cells which is able to produce local itching and swelling.

Immunoglobulins: An antibody molecule produced by white cells. There are five sorts, IgG, IgM, IgA, IgD and IgE.

Ion: A single positive or negative atom or molecule. The charge is caused by the gain or loss of an electron.

Ionizing and Non-ionization (NIR): Ionizing radiation has sufficient energy to ionize (remove an electron from the outer shell) of an atom or molecule. It becomes ionizing radiation when its wavelength becomes less than 4×10^{-7} m. Non-ionization has a wavelength of greater than 4×10^{-7} m but may still cause health problems.

Magnetic field: A magnetic field is induced when an electric charge is in steady motion. The units of magnetic fields are Teslas (1 microTesla = 0.8 ampere per metre). The earth's magnetic field is equivalent to 50 microTeslas.

Masking: A basic phenomenon of allergy in which you initially feel better when you are exposed to a neotoxin to which you are allergic. It is due to adaption of enzymes. The process of masking is later followed by unmasking.

Mast cell: A cell containing histamine granules and carrying IgE molecules on its surface.

	Histamine is released when the IgE is triggered by an antigen it recognizes.
Neotoxin:	A very broad term used to describe any sort of harmful agent which may cause an environmentally induced illness, often called an 'allergy', in a susceptible individual. Potential sources of neotoxin are biological, chemical, physical and mental.
Piezoelectric:	Some crystals produce an electric voltage when they are compressed or twisted. Equally applying a voltage to two surfaces will cause a change in shape of the crystals.
Placebo:	A tablet with no active ingredient. Some patients will get better when given placebo with no active ingredient.
Prostaglandins:	Very important substances, derived from fatty acids, which may act locally to cause inflammation.
Proteins:	Molecules with a molecular weight above 10,000, which are an essential constituent of all living cells. Proteins have three dimensional structures which are often essential for their enzymatic abilities.
Provocation – neutralization:	This is an important phenomenon in allergy. Small amounts of a neotoxin placed in the mouth, on the skin, or injected into the skin have the power to provoke allergic symptoms. These symptoms may be turned off or neutralized by a more dilute micro- dose. This technique has been used successfully to treat food, and chemical allergies and also some viral infections.
Quantum:	Energy occurs in tiny packages (each one called a quantum). The higher the frequency, the greater the size of each quantum of energy.
Rhinitis:	Inflammation of the mucus membrane lining the inside of the nose.
Schumann radiation:	A naturally occurring ELF radiation of between 7 and 30 Hertz. It is caused by the conducting earth and iono- sphere acting as a resonator with the non-conducting atmosphere in between. The resonator is energized by thunderstorms around the world.
Sensitization:	An allergen stimulates an allergic reaction by sensitizing the body. Sensitization can occur at any exposure after the first.
Spreading Phenomenon:	A basic phenomenon in allergy where the body be- comes sensitive to more and more neotoxins. This is a common phenomenon with chemicals.
Steroids:	Also known as corticosteroids, steroids are hormones pro- duced by the adrenal cortex. They have many functions and effects on metabolism, including stopping inflamma- tion and allergic reactions.
Systemic:	Affecting the whole body.
Unmasking:	A basic phenomenon in allergy that follows masking.

During unmasking the enzymes initially produced in response to the neotoxin lose their activity.

Topical: Local action when a substance is applied directly to a single part of the body.

Urticaria: An allergic reaction visible in the skin caused by the effect of histamine. The characteristic signs are swelling, redness and itching.

Wavelength: The distance between two successive peaks of a wave, usually given in metres. The wavelength is inversely proportional to the frequency.

USEFUL ADDRESSES

Addresses and telephone numbers given below are correct at time of going to press. If you require information, don't forget to send a large stamped self-addressed envelope.

Action Against Allergy
43 The Downs
London SW20 8HG
Tel: 081 947 5082

An allergy education organization

Action for Research into Multiple Sclerosis
11 Dartmouth St
London SW1H 9BL
Tel: 071 222 3224

Interested in finding a cure for multiple sclerosis

Allergy Support Group and Hyperactive Children's Support Group
Mrs N Knowles
11 The Paddox
Squitchley Lane
Oxford OX2 7PN
Tel: 0865 52824

An allergy support group

American Academy of Environmental Medicine
1750 Humboldt St
Denver
Colorado 80218
USA

The association for American Physicians who practise Environmental Medicine.

ASH (Action on Smoking and Health)
5–11 Mortimer St
London W1N 7RH
Tel: 071 637 9843

A pressure group to reduce tobacco consumption

Asthma and Allergy Treatment and Research Centre
12 Vernon St
Derby DE1 1FT
Tel: 0332 362461

An allergy research organization particularly interested in hay fever and asthma

Asthma Research Council
12–14 Pembridge Square
London
Tel: 071 226 2260

An organization interested in research into the cause and cures for asthma

Asthma Society and Friends of the Asthma Research Council
300 Upper St
London N1 2XX
Tel: 071 226 2260

An organization interested in research into the cause and cures for asthma

Biolab
The Stone House
9 Weymouth St
London W1N 3FF
Tel: 071 636 5959/5905

Allergy laboratories carrying out hair, sweat, mineral, vitamins and pesticides analysis

Breakspear Hospital (Allergy and Environmental Medicine)
Medical Director: Dr Jean Monro
High St
Abbots Langley
Hertfordshire WD4 9HT
Tel: 0923 261333

Britain's only fully equipped allergy hospital

British Dyslexia Association
Church Lane
Peppard
Oxfordshire RG9 5JN

An association interested in finding answers to dyslexia

British Holistic Medical Association
179 Gloucester Place
London NW1 6DX
Tel: 071 262 5299

An organization of doctors, other practitioners and public interested in holistic medicine.

British Migraine Association
Evergreen
Ottermead Lane
Ottershaw
Chertsey
Surrey

An association interested in finding cures for migraine

British Migraine Society
178A High Rd
Byfleet
Weybridge
Surrey KT14 7ED
Tel: 09323 52468

An organization interested in finding cures for migraine

British Society for Allergy and Environmental Medicine (BSAEM)
'Acorns'
Romsey Road
Southampton SO4 2NN

A society for doctors interested in Environmental Medicine

British Society for Nutritional Medicine
5 Somerhill Road
Hove
East Sussex BN3 1RP

A society interested in the effects of food on health

Coeliac Society
PO Box 220
High Wycombe
Buckinghamshire HP11 2HY

A society to help sufferers of coeliac disease

College of Health
18 Victoria Park Square
London E2 9PF
Tel: 081 6263

An organization interested in helping patients receive better healthcare

Cotton On
29 North Clifton St
Lytham FY8 5HW
Tel: 0253 736611

Suppliers of cotton clothing

Council for Environmental Education (CEE)
School of Education
University of Reading
London Road
Reading RG1 5AQ
Tel: 0734-318921

An organization interested in further education about environmental matters.

Environmental Medicine Foundation (EMF)
Symondsbury House
Bridport
Dorset DT6 6HB
Tel: 0308 22956

A registered charity that organizes Environmental Medicine research

Foresight
The Old Vicarage
Witley
Godalming
Surrey GU8 5PN
Tel: 042879 4500

An organization that educates and arranges pre-conceptual care.

Friends of the Earth (FoE)
26–28 Underwood St
London N1 7JQ
Tel: 071-490-1555

A campaigning organization devoted to reducing pollution

Friends of the Earth (Scotland)
15 Windsor St
Edinburgh EH7 5LA
Tel: 031-557-3432

A campaigning organization devoted to reducing pollution

Henry Doubleday Research Association (HDRA)
Ryton-on-Dunsmore
Coventry CV8 3LG
Tel: 0203-303517

National centre for organic gardening

Human Ecology Foundation (Toronto)
R R 1
Goodwood
Ontario
Canada LOC 1AO

To promote interest in Environmental Medicine

The Human Ecology Research Foundation
505 North Lake Shore Drive
Suite 6506
Chicago
Illinois 60611
USA

An organization researching into Environmental Medicine

Hyperactive Childrens Support Group
59 Meadowside
Angmering
Littlehampton
West Sussex BN16 4BW
Tel: 0903 725 182

A support organization for parents with hyperactive children

The Institute of Biophysical Medicine
20 Coppice Walk
Cheswick Green
Solihull B90 4HY
Tel: 05646 2186

An organization for research into the effects of electromagnetic radiation on health

Institute for Complementary Medicine
21 Portland Place
London W1N 3AF
Tel: 071 636 0543

An organization interested in all forms of complementary medicine

Irish Allergy Association
PO Box 1067
Churchtown
Dublin 14

An organization to promote interest in allergy

Larkhill Laboratories
225 Putney Bridge Road
London SW15 2PY

Laboratories carrying out allergy tests

McCarrison Society
76 Harley St
London W1N 1AE
Tel: 071 935 3925

A society to study the relationships between nutrition and health

Medic Alert Foundation
11–13 Clifton Terrace
London N4 3JP
Tel: 071 263 8596

An organization that keeps details of patients allergies on file for emergency access.

Medisoft
148 Highfield Road
Hall Green
Birmingham
Tel: 0212 702 2688

The computer software house responsible for the 'CADTEMP' program

Myalgic Encephalomyelitis (ME)
The Moss
Third Avenue
Stanford-le-Hope
Essex SS17 8EL

An organization to help sufferers from ME

National Association for Colitis and Crohn's Disease
98A London Road
St Albans
Herts AL1 1NX
Tel: 9727 44296

An organization to help patients suffering from inflammatory bowel disorders

National Association for Research into Allergies
PO Box 45
Hinckley
Leicester LE10 1JY

An organization interested in encouraging research into allergy

National Childbirth Trust
9 Queensborough Terrace
London W2
Tel: 071 221 3833

An organization interested in empowering women to have the type of delivery they wish.

National Eczema Society
Tavistock House North
Tavistock Square
London WC1H 9SR
Tel: 071 388 4097

An organization to help sufferers from eczema

National Pure Water Association
Bank Farm
Aston Pigott
Westbury
Shrewsbury ST5 9HH
Tel: 0784 383 445

An organization interested in the quality of water

National Society for Clean Air (NSCA)
136 North St
Brighton BN1 1RG
Tel: 0273 26313

An organization interested in the quality of air

Dr Mark Payne
20 Coppice Walk
Cheswick Green
Solihull
W Midlands B90 4HY
Tel: 05646 2186

Author and Broadcaster

Sanity
77 Moss Lane
Pinner
Middlesex

An organization interested in finding nutritional and biochemical reasons and cures for mental illness

Schizophrenia Association of Gt Britain
Bryn Hyfryd
The Crescent
Bangor
Gwynedd LL57 2AG
Tel: 0248 354048

An organization to help sufferers from schizophrenia

The Soil Association
86–88 Colston Street
Bristol BS1 5BB
Tel: 0272 290661

An organization that warrants the safety of organic produce

Vegan Society
7 Battle Road
St Leonards on Sea
East Sussex TN37 7AA
Tel: 0424 427393

An organization for vegans

Vegetarian Society
Parkdale
Dunham Rd
Altrincham
Cheshire WA14 4QG
Tel: 061 928 0793

An organization for vegetarians

INDEX

Of further interest:

SHIATSU:
The Complete Guide
Chris Jarmey and Gabriel Mojay

The definitive Shiatsu guide and reference for the beginner, student and practitioner of this increasingly popular therapy, and for anyone with a serious interest in bodywork. Beginning with a brief history of Shiatsu, the authors then explain:

- the concept of Ki, the power which unifies and animates

- the essential elements of competent Shiatsu

- the use of hands, palms, thumbs, fingers, forearms, knees, feet and breathing

- the Channels as they are used in Shiatsu

- the basic treatment techniques

- Shiatsu therapy and Traditional Oriental Medicine

- the various forms of traditional Oriental diagnosis

- the Five Elements and Hara focus

Illustrated throughout and going deeply into the subject both in a general and spiritual context, *Shiatsu* is the indispensable guide.

THE CALM TECHNIQUE:
Simple Meditation Methods that Really Work

Paul Wilson

Close your eyes and you will see clearly
Cease to listen and you will hear truth
TAOIST POEM

Of all the techniques to enhance health, happiness and harmony, meditation is one of the most effective and easy to learn. This practical introduction explains:

● the nature of meditation

● the nature of the stress problems meditation can solve

● a step-by-step guide to how to meditate

The author has also included a variety of exercises, and a question and answer section, as well as some tips on other lifestyle techniques to enhance the effectiveness of meditation. Simply by giving yourself 30 minutes a day, you will be able to ease stress, improve your sex-life, and generate self-confidence.

ESSENTIAL SUPPLEMENTS FOR WOMEN
What every woman should know about vitamins, minerals, enzymes and amino acids

Carolyn Reuben and Dr Joan Priestley

At last a guide specially for women that explains how vitamin and mineral supplements are useful for treating common female ailments, for preventing and even combating major disease, and for enhancing and maintaining good health.

Begins with every woman's health concerns – from menstruation to menopause – and tells you the vitamins, minerals and amino acids that are helpful for the particular condition.

Also contains information on the most suitable dosages for each supplement for the specific health purpose, and includes many case histories of women who have successfully used supplements to promote good health and fight disease.

SHIATSU	0 7225 2243 6	£14.99
THE CALM TECHNIQUE	0 7225 1468 9	£3.99
ESSENTIAL SUPPLEMENTS FOR WOMEN	0 7225 2429 3	£6.99
THE BIORHYTHM LIFE-PLANNER	0 7225 2515 X	£7.99
MEDAU: THE ART OF ENERGY	0 7225 2572 9	£6.99
AUTOGENIC TRAINING	0 7225 2616 4	£8.99
LET'S GET WELL	0 7225 2701 2	£5.99
BODYFIT	0 7225 2691 1	£7.99

All these books are available at your local bookseller or can be ordered direct from the publishers.

To order direct just tick the titles you want and fill in the form below:

Name: ....

Address: ....

....

....Postcode:.............................

Send to: Thorsons Mail Order, Dept 31, HarperCollins*Publishers*, Westerhill Road, Bishopbriggs, Glasgow G64 2QT.
Please enclose a cheque or postal order or debit my Visa/Access account –

Credit card no: ....

Expiry date: ....

Signature: ....

– to the value of the cover price plus:

UK & BFPO: Add £1.00 for the first book and 25p for each additional book ordered.

Overseas orders including Eire: Please add £2.95 service charge. Books will be sent by surface mail but quotes for airmail despatches will be given on request.

24 HOUR TELEPHONE ORDERING SERVICE FOR ACCESS/VISA CARDHOLDERS – TEL: **041 772 2281.**